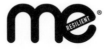

A RESILIENCE AND GRATITUDE JOURNAL
BY AWESOME INC®

*Life is full of wonder
if you only stop and look.*

WWW.THEAWESOMEINC.CO.NZ (NZ/AU)
WWW.THEAWESOMEINC.COM (USA)

RESILIENT ME® GRATITUDE JOURNAL BY AWESOME INC®
BUILDING RESILIENCE & BOOSTING HAPPINESS

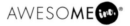

Published by ME Incorporated Limited T/A AwesoME Inc®
PO Box 95158, Swanson, Auckland 0653, New Zealand

First edition published in 2018. This edition published 2021.

WWW.THEAWESOMEINC.CO.NZ (NZ/AU)
WWW.THEAWESOMEINC.COM (USA)

Contents

Learn to become stronger and wiser through the experiences of everyday life.

Resilience is more than putting on a brave face. It's coming through adversity positively, and using what we learn to strengthen us. It's hard to know where to begin when anxieties are pitching in from all angles, that's where we can help you. This journal is your starting point to create a healthier, happier you.

The Resilient ME® journal is filled with practical tools and techniques that are easy to follow, based on the science of positive psychology. You can learn to build your resilience, boost your happiness, improve your health and well-being, and rebuild your life.

STAY FOCUSED. KEEP CALM. BE POSITIVE.

Humans are predisposed to see and focus on what goes wrong in our lives, to see the danger, so we can protect ourselves. It is called 'negative bias' and it is how we have survived. But it also has the added effect of making us feel like we aren't enough, or that we don't have enough, or that only bad things happen to us. We feel stressed and unhappy, even though there are a lot of positive things in our lives. There are many ways we can interrupt this bias, to rewire our brains to focus on the good things, to think more clearly, and in turn increase our life satisfaction, so we feel more content, and happy. One of the most effective ways to do this is by practising gratitude.

If this is your first AwesoME Inc® journal you will find tips on page 12 about how to get the most out of using a gratitude journal, and examples on page eight and nine. We recommend you keep your journal somewhere you will see it every day, as a gentle reminder to fill it in, like beside your bed or on your desk. The pages of this journal are not dated as we believe that filling in your journal should be something you do when it is right for you. Do not feel guilty if you have missed days; feel grateful that you have picked it up and filled it in. This journal will become a very precious book in the future because as you fill it in you will be able to look back and read all the amazing things that have happened in your life.

Gratitude is one of the powerful tools you can use to transform your life to one that is fulfilling, and a lot less chaotic. You will realise that the most important things in life, the ones we become truly grateful for, are the simple things. With this realisation you can release a lot of stress from your life. Gratitude is not about avoiding negative experiences altogether, it is about training your brain to appreciate the positive experiences when they happen and taking the time to focus on them.

You already possess everything necessary to become great.

Try to focus some of your gratitude on areas in your life that are lacking in fulfillment. For example, maybe a relationship that has love at its core seems to be a bit lost? By looking for the good in that relationship or situation you will start to see more good and feel more warmth towards the other person. It can be hard at the start but the more you try the easier it will become.

Write regularly and consistently if you can, whether you write everyday or once a week, make a commitment to yourself. Be specific about what you are grateful for – elaborating in detail about a particular person or thing carries many more benefits than a superficial list of many things.

We all wish to be happy, and want that for our loved ones as well. Being happy all the time is not achievable, but having a content and fulfilling life speckled with lots of happiness is. Using gratitude helps you to see things in a new light, you will start to see the good things, rather than focusing and dwelling on the hassles. The benefits to you will be numerous.

Scientists are discovering a host of benefits that practising gratitude can bring you, including a stronger immune system, lower blood pressure, higher levels of positive emotions, more joy, optimism and happiness. You will feel more generosity and compassion towards others, feel less lonely and isolated, and can experience decreased symptoms of depression and anxiety.* These are just some of the amazing benefits that can be achieved by using gratitude daily; turn to page ten to find out more. We are sure you will start to notice a positive effect once you start filling out this book.

RESILIENCE STARTS HERE...

The Resilient ME® journal is more than a gratitude journal – it is also a resilience building tool. When crisis hits having skills that build up your resilience can be a life-saver. Helping yourself and those you love survive through difficult times can seem like a distant dream. Imagine not just surviving but thriving, and becoming stronger and wiser through the experiences of everyday life. That is what building resilience is all about, and in this journal you will find added tools and techniques, based on the latest scientific research, to help you do just that. Read through the pages and fill in the activities to learn amazing yet simple ways you can build your emotional resilience.

Gratitude, breathing and meditation, mindfulness, managing emotions, creating meaningful connections and a positive mindset, self-care, exercise, sleep and nutrition, are all ways you can build resilience and help you to stay focused, to think clearly, and to remain calm in the face of adversity.

Resilience isn't about a "stiff upper lip" or just battling through. It's about having the skills to help you remain calm and positive, growing and learning rather than feeling swamped, and seeing the situation for what it is. Just because you're the grown-up doesn't mean you've got it together. Being an adult today can be overwhelming. Dealing with work, home-life, partners, kids, pets, financial worries, world-troubles. It's hard to know where to start, so start with this journal.

*Research by Prof. Robert Emmons, The University of California & Prof. Michael McCullough, University of Miami

Remember to be gentle with yourself, you have a whole lot happening. Take a moment to pause and breathe. In this fast-paced, stressful world, you need to find ways to be silent and find calm within yourself. How can you really know what you feel, and who you are, if you never stop and listen? Explore the pages of this journal and use the tools and techniques to turn stress into positive energy, and use it to push yourself towards your goals and dreams.

The words 'THANK YOU!' have been included on each journal page to remind you to say thank you as much as you can each day. You will also find inspirational words, to lift your spirit so you can see just how miraculous you really are. There are also personal challenges and acts of kindness to complete to help you connect with yourself and others.

There is a happiness scale on the edge of the page, make sure to colour this in as it will be a great visual tool to see how you have been feeling when you flip back through the pages. There is also space to write your word for the day. Are you feeling focused, strong, connected, or upset, anxious, angry? Use this, the happiness scale and the healthy habit tracker to spot patterns between your mood, quality of sleep, exercise, relaxation and connections. You might be surprised!

At the bottom of each page is a space for your daily positive affirmation, or your strengths. Here you simply write what you want to manifest about yourself or life. You might not be a calm person right now, but want to be, so write 'I AM CALM'. You are then affirming to yourself that you ARE calm. Other examples: *I am confident; I am healthy; I am successful; I am wealthy, I am amazing!*

Thank you so much for joining with us and including this journal as part of your life. We wish happiness and contentment for you and for all those around you.

THE AWESOME INC® TEAM
BUILDING RESILIENCE & BOOSTING HAPPINESS

PERSONAL CHALLENGE
Laugh today – as much as you can.

20/11/20

DATE

↑

Undated so you don't feel
guilty when you miss days.

↑

inspiration/motivation/challenge
for the day.

TODAY I AM GRATEFUL FOR...

A quiet moment in the sunshine to drink my cup of coffee,

it was nice to have a peaceful moment to reflect.

Our warm home full of food and money to pay for it !

The great conversation with my workmate, it made

me feel better about a difficult situation. ↑

Use this space to list three to five things
you are grateful for today. An event,
experience, person or thing in your life.

HAPPINESS SCALE (%)

100 · 75 · 50 · 25 · 0

← Use these tools to spot patterns
between your mood and habits.

Thank You! Thank You! Thank You! Thank You! Thank You! Thank You!

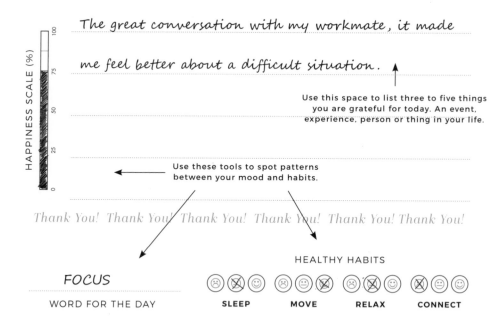

FOCUS

WORD FOR THE DAY

HEALTHY HABITS

| SLEEP | MOVE | RELAX | CONNECT |

I AM

POSITIVE AFFIRMATIONS

I am happy, healthy, successful and full of

abundance.

↑
What are your heart's desires?
The Universe is listening.

23/11/20

INSPIRATION
*Retrain your mind to see
the good in everything.*

WHAT WENT RIGHT THIS WEEK....

I had a clear run of traffic to the office and found a

car park easily, it started my day off great!

My boss acknowledged all the hard work I put in last week,

it made me feel appreciated.

I remembered to sign up the kids to their holiday

programme, they will be so happy.

How would you rate
your happiness/mood today? →

HAPPINESS SCALE (%)

Use this space to record positive things
that happened in your week, to tune into
the sources of goodness in your life.

Choose one word that describes
your day. Or that you choose to
focus on today.

Thank You! Thank You! Thank You! Thank You! Thank You! Thank You!

HEALTHY HABITS

SLEEP   MOVE   RELAX   CONNECT

Track your quality of sleep,
exercise, meditation and
meaningful connections.

CHALLENGING

WORD FOR THE DAY

MY STRENGTHS

I am confident, optimistic, resilient and motivated.

Focus on your strengths, not your flaws.
What would you like them to be?

9

Why gratitude works

Gratitude is an easy and effective way of retraining your brain and is strongly and consistently associated with greater happiness.

IMPROVES MENTAL HEALTH

Challenging negative thought patterns helps to calm the anxious, and boost the moods of those who are depressed. Practising gratitude floods the brain with positive chemicals and sparks brain activity critical to sleep, orgasms, mood regulation and metabolism.

IMPROVES PHYSICAL HEALTH

Strengthens the immune system, lowers blood pressure, reduces symptoms of illness, and makes you less bothered by aches and pains. Practising gratitude also helps to shift the heart rhythm and thereby increases the coherence of body functions, which facilitates higher cognitive functions, creating emotional stability and a state of calm.

INCREASES RESILIENCE

Helps you bounce back from stressful events and helps you deal with adversity by acting as a buffer against internalising symptoms.

INCREASES SOCIAL CONNECTION

Feelings of gratitude for others can help you feel a greater connection, and feel more satisfied, with friends, family, school, community and yourself. Gratitude builds compassion and empathy – the more thankful we feel, the more likely we are to act pro-socially toward others, causing them to feel grateful and setting up a beautiful virtuous cascade.

INCREASES PRODUCTIVITY

Showing gratitude to others makes them feel inspired and uplifted – these feelings of elevation bolster motivation to become healthier, more generous people, but also better, more productive workers.

Based on research by: R. Emmons, The University of California, USA; M. Mcculough, University of Miami, USA; P. J. Mills, The University of California, USA; R. Zahn, National Institutes of Health, Cognitive Neuroscience Section, USA & The University of Manchester, UK; P. Kini, Indiana University, USA; E. Simon-Thomas, The Greater Good Science Center, UC Berkeley, USA; J. Froh, Hofstra University, USA; M. A. Stoeckel, American University, USA; A. Wood, University of Stirling, UK; Institute of HeartMath, USA.

NEVER GIVE UP, TODAY IS A NEW DAY, A NEW CHANCE.

inspiration

The habit of being grateful starts with appreciating every good thing in life, and recognising that there is nothing too small for you to be thankful for.

USE THESE TIPS TO START YOUR GRATITUDE PRACTICE...

WRITE REGULARLY AND CONSISTENTLY

A good amount is three or four times a week. Evidence suggests writing occasionally is more beneficial than daily journaling because you can adapt to positive events, and become numb to them.

BE SPECIFIC ABOUT WHAT YOU ARE GRATEFUL FOR

Elaborating in detail about a particular person or thing carries many more benefits than just a list of things. For example: "I am grateful for water and sunshine." Instead you could write: "I am grateful for water, because it fuels me" "I am grateful for sunshine because it makes me feel happy and warm."

SAVOUR SURPRISES

Record events that were unexpected or surprising. Be grateful that you avoided a negative outcome, and don't take good fortune for granted.

KEEP THE NEGATIVE OUT

Make it a purely positive-only exercise. The brain has a weird way of focusing on the negative; for example instead of saying " I am grateful that I didn't miss the bus this morning." try " I am grateful that I was early for the bus this morning."

DON'T WAIT FOR THE RIGHT TIME

Some people like a routine, but if you have an awesome experience write it down straight away.

THINK OF WHAT MATERIAL POSSESSIONS ALLOW YOU TO DO

An example of this might be you are grateful that you have a car, but it is so much more powerful to recognise what having a car allows you to do, or experience.

FOCUS ON PEOPLE

Each time other people help us they are doing so on purpose, it is called intention. They give something up to help us, such as their time or energy. Try recognising the personal cost to them when they help you, and acknowledge the benefit to you .

> NOTICING MORE AND MORE WHAT WE
> CAN BE GRATEFUL FOR HELPS US TO REALISE THAT
> HAPPINESS IS RIGHT HERE WITHIN US.

WRITE ABOUT SITUATIONS AND EXPERIENCES

Remember a good event, experience, person or thing in your life and the emotions that go with it. Re-imagining a positive feeling is a powerful tool that can increase coherence of the brain, and heart, creating emotional stability, and facilitating a state of calm.

REVISE AND REPEAT

If you find yourself writing the same things that is OK, but try to hone in on a different detail each time.

CONSIDER LIFE WITHOUT

Try imagining what your life would be like without certain people or things. Write down how they help you.

COUNT YOUR GIFTS

Thinking of the good things in your life as gifts helps you to not take them for granted. Try to relish and savour the gifts you've received.

What makes me happy?

Identify things, people or activities that make you happy. Come back to this page when you are feeling sad, for ideas on flipping your mood.

THINGS I AM GRATEFUL FOR ABOUT ME...

THINGS I AM GRATEFUL TO HAVE IN MY LIFE...

ACT OF KINDNESS
*Cook a meal for someone
who needs a break.*

TODAY I AM GRATEFUL FOR...

HAPPINESS SCALE (%)

100

75

50

25

0

Thank You! Thank You! Thank You! Thank You! Thank You! Thank You!

HEALTHY HABITS

SLEEP   **MOVE**   **RELAX**   **CONNECT**

WORD FOR THE DAY

POSITIVE AFFIRMATIONS

I
AM

*Don't be afraid to be who you are
authentically meant to be.*

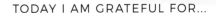

DATE

TODAY I AM GRATEFUL FOR...

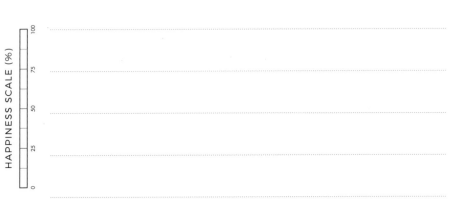

HAPPINESS SCALE (%)

100

75

50

25

0

Thank You! Thank You! Thank You! Thank You! Thank You! Thank You!

HEALTHY HABITS

WORD FOR THE DAY

☹ 😐 😊   ☹ 😐 😊   ☹ 😐 😊   ☹ 😐 😊

SLEEP   **MOVE**   **RELAX**   **CONNECT**

I
AM

POSITIVE AFFIRMATIONS

Enough is all you need.

TODAY I AM GRATEFUL FOR...

HAPPINESS SCALE (%)

100

75

50

25

0

Thank You! Thank You! Thank You! Thank You! Thank You! Thank You!

HEALTHY HABITS

SLEEP   **MOVE**   **RELAX**   **CONNECT**

WORD FOR THE DAY

POSITIVE AFFIRMATIONS

I AM

DATE

TODODAY I AM GRATEFUL FOR...

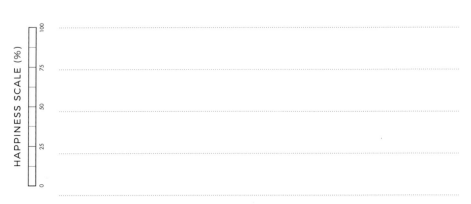

HAPPINESS SCALE (%)

100

75

50

25

0

Thank You! Thank You! Thank You! Thank You! Thank You! Thank You!

HEALTHY HABITS

WORD FOR THE DAY

SLEEP   **MOVE**   **RELAX**   **CONNECT**

I
AM

POSITIVE AFFIRMATIONS

DATE

Don't waste today thinking about
what happened yesterday.

WHAT WENT RIGHT THIS WEEK....

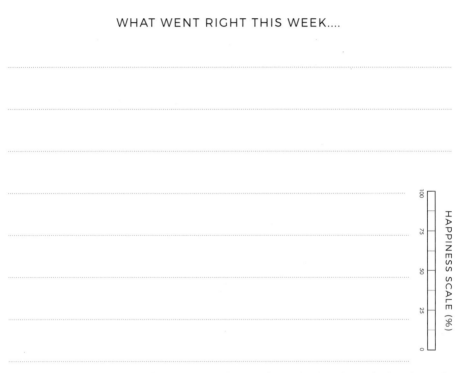

HAPPINESS SCALE (%)

100
75
50
25
0

Thank You! Thank You! Thank You! Thank You! Thank You! Thank You!

HEALTHY HABITS

SLEEP   **MOVE**   **RELAX**   **CONNECT**

WORD FOR THE DAY

MY STRENGTHS

*Life is too short to not be
happy as much as we can be.*

....
DATE

TODAY I AM GRATEFUL FOR...

HAPPINESS SCALE (%)

100

75

50

25

0

Thank You! Thank You! Thank You! Thank You! Thank You! Thank You!

HEALTHY HABITS

WORD FOR THE DAY

SLEEP   **MOVE**   **RELAX**   **CONNECT**

I AM

POSITIVE AFFIRMATIONS

The greatest work you will
do is the inner work on you.

TODAY I AM GRATEFUL FOR...

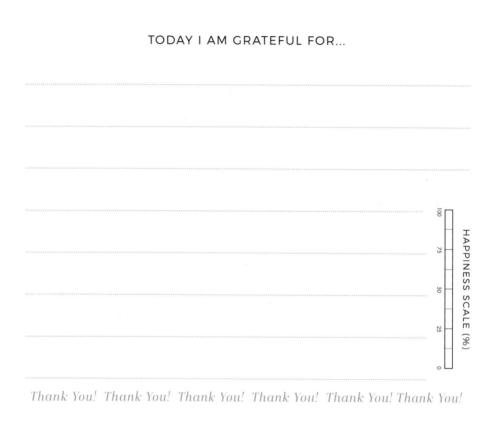

HAPPINESS SCALE (%)

100

75

50

25

0

Thank You! Thank You! Thank You! Thank You! Thank You! Thank You!

HEALTHY HABITS

SLEEP   **MOVE**   **RELAX**   **CONNECT**

WORD FOR THE DAY

POSITIVE AFFIRMATIONS

I
AM

Great peace can be found within
if you learn to quiet your mind.

DATE

TODAY I AM GRATEFUL FOR...

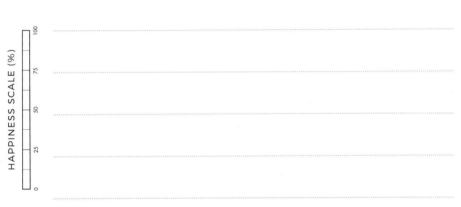

HAPPINESS SCALE (%)

100

75

50

25

0

Thank You! Thank You! Thank You! Thank You! Thank You! Thank You!

HEALTHY HABITS

SLEEP   MOVE   RELAX   CONNECT

WORD FOR THE DAY

I
AM

POSITIVE AFFIRMATIONS

Go for a walk and notice
the earth around you.

DATE

TODAY I AM GRATEFUL FOR...

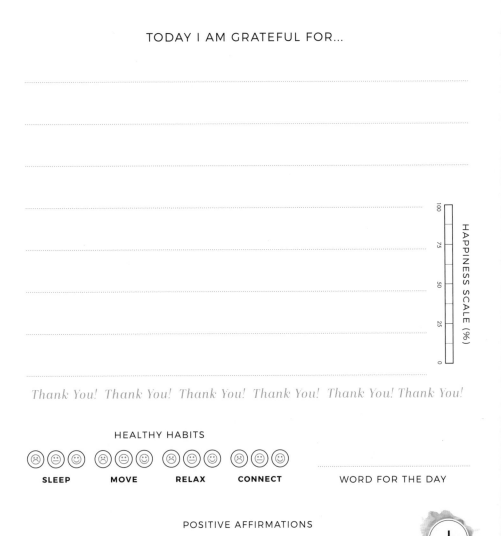

HAPPINESS SCALE (%)

100

75

50

25

0

Thank You! Thank You! Thank You! Thank You! Thank You! Thank You!

HEALTHY HABITS

SLEEP   **MOVE**   **RELAX**   **CONNECT**

WORD FOR THE DAY

POSITIVE AFFIRMATIONS

I AM

Do it now! Sometimes later becomes never.

DATE

WHAT WENT RIGHT THIS WEEK....

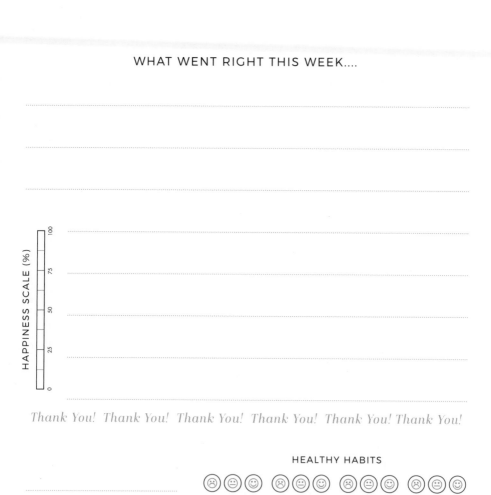

HAPPINESS SCALE (%)

100

75

50

25

0

Thank You! Thank You! Thank You! Thank You! Thank You! Thank You!

HEALTHY HABITS

WORD FOR THE DAY

SLEEP   **MOVE**   **RELAX**   **CONNECT**

MY STRENGTHS

....
DATE

TODAY I AM GRATEFUL FOR...

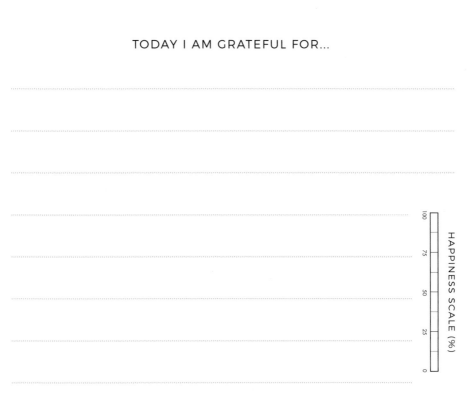

HAPPINESS SCALE (%)

100
75
50
25
0

Thank You! Thank You! Thank You! Thank You! Thank You! Thank You!

HEALTHY HABITS

SLEEP   **MOVE**   **RELAX**   **CONNECT**

WORD FOR THE DAY

POSITIVE AFFIRMATIONS

I
AM

25

Trust the Universe.

DATE

TODAY I AM GRATEFUL FOR...

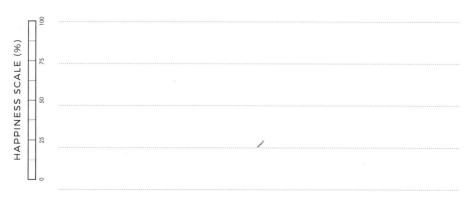

HAPPINESS SCALE (%)

100

75

50

25

0

Thank You! Thank You! Thank You! Thank You! Thank You! Thank You!

HEALTHY HABITS

WORD FOR THE DAY

SLEEP **MOVE** **RELAX** **CONNECT**

I AM

POSITIVE AFFIRMATIONS

What is this life for but to enjoy love in all its forms.

....
DATE

TODAY I AM GRATEFUL FOR...

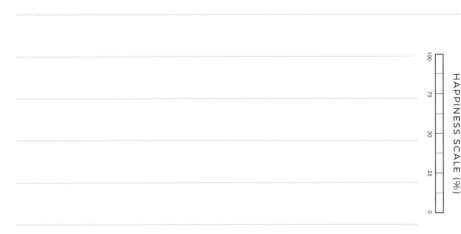

HAPPINESS SCALE (%)

100

75

50

25

0

Thank You! Thank You! Thank You! Thank You! Thank You! Thank You!

HEALTHY HABITS

SLEEP   **MOVE**   **RELAX**   **CONNECT**

WORD FOR THE DAY

POSITIVE AFFIRMATIONS

I AM

*Be conscious of what you eat today
and try and crowd in as many
wholefoods as possible.*

DATE

TODAY I AM GRATEFUL FOR...

HAPPINESS SCALE (%)

100

75

50

25

0

Thank You! Thank You! Thank You! Thank You! Thank You! Thank You!

HEALTHY HABITS

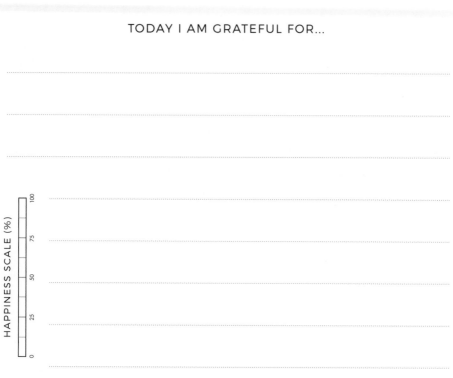

WORD FOR THE DAY

SLEEP   MOVE   RELAX   CONNECT

I
AM

POSITIVE AFFIRMATIONS

Sometimes through the hardest of experiences we can find the magic within.

WHAT WENT RIGHT THIS WEEK....

HAPPINESS SCALE (%)

100

75

50

25

0

Thank You! Thank You! Thank You! Thank You! Thank You! Thank You!

HEALTHY HABITS

SLEEP   **MOVE**   **RELAX**   **CONNECT**

WORD FOR THE DAY

MY STRENGTHS

Love is at our very core,
remember to let it shine out.

TODAY I AM GRATEFUL FOR...

HAPPINESS SCALE (%)

100

75

50

25

0

Thank You! Thank You! Thank You! Thank You! Thank You! Thank You!

HEALTHY HABITS

WORD FOR THE DAY

SLEEP　　**MOVE**　　**RELAX**　　**CONNECT**

I
AM

POSITIVE AFFIRMATIONS

I AM ENOUGH...

SMART ENOUGH

WORTHY ENOUGH

STRONG ENOUGH

CONFIDENT ENOUGH

UNIQUE ENOUGH

PRECIOUS ENOUGH

inspiration

40 ways to boost your mood

We all have days that overwhelm, when everything just seems all too much, and your mood takes you down even further. Use these simple tips for self-care to boost your mood and help you feel better. We are more resilient, and able to handle life's stress, when we are feeling our best both physically and emotionally.

DO SOME COLOURING IN OR DOODLING

TAKE A SHOWER OR BATH

DRINK A GLASS OF WATER

READ A BOOK
Increase your knowledge and feel inspired.

WALK BAREFOOT ON THE GRASS

GO TO BED EARLY

ASK FOR A HUG
Pets love hugs too!

DANCE LIKE NO-ONE IS WATCHING

MAKE YOUR BED

TAKE A COFFEE BREAK

PAMPER YOURSELF
Get a massage, manicure or get your hair done.

DO SOMETHING PRODUCTIVE
Clean, organise your desk, write a to-do-list that is easily accomplished.

SAY 'I LOVE YOU' IN THE MIRROR

FOCUS ON SOMETHING THAT MAKES YOU HAPPY

CHANGE YOUR ENVIRONMENT

BRING NATURE INSIDE
Buy yourself some flowers.

DIFFUSE ESSENTIAL OILS
Use scents like orange or lavender that promote calm.

TALK TO A FRIEND

CREATE A VISION BOARD

WATCH A
FUNNY MOVIE

DO SOMETHING
NICE FOR SOMEONE
Giving produces endorphins in the brain
often called 'helpers high'.

DO SOME EXERCISE
It will boost your energy and self esteem,
relieve stress and improve sleep.

SPEND TIME
IN SILENCE

WEAR YOUR
FAVOURITE
OUTFIT

DO A
MINDFULNESS EXERCISE
Lay on your back and look at the clouds,
listen to the sounds around you.

HAVE LUNCH
WITH A FRIEND

GET UP AND
STRETCH

TURN OFF
SOCIAL MEDIA

SIT IN
NATURE

ENTERTAIN YOURSELF
Go to the movies or spend time
on a favourite hobby.

VISUALISE SOMETHING
OR SOMEONE YOU LOVE
Concentrate on your breathing too
and feel your heart rate slow down.

WRITE IN
THIS JOURNAL

WRITE A
LETTER TO
A FRIEND

HAVE A
HEALTHY MEAL
OR SNACK

SIT IN
THE SUN

TURN OFF
ALL ELECTRONICS

GO FOR A WALK
The change in location will take
your mind off your troubles.

DO SOME
YOGA

LISTEN TO
UPBEAT MUSIC

HOST A
PARTY

TAKE SOME
DEEP BELLY
BREATHS

DO SOME
MEDITATION

DO
SOMETHING
NEW

Negative emotions are often the hardest to deal with, but they are just as much a part of life as the positive ones.

MANAGING EMOTIONS

Do you ever feel like your life is an emotional rollercoaster? In the course of one day you can experience a range of emotions, from happiness to anxiety, anger to excitement. You name it, you can feel it. It is really important to remember that ALL emotions are normal, even the negative ones like sadness and anger, and are needed to lead a healthy life. You need to learn to deal with the bad as well as the good, and cope with it all so you can live your happiest life. Instead of holding onto those emotions that make you feel bad, you must remember they will pass. Try this:

STEP 1:	**STEP 2:**	**STEP 3:**
NOTICE WHAT EMOTION YOU ARE FEELING	NAME AND ACKNOWLEDGE THE EMOTION	TAKE A DEEP BREATH AND LET IT PASS

HOW DOES IT WORK?

Naming or labeling emotions reduces the power of that feeling by bridging the gap between thoughts and feelings. Some research* has found that when emotional experience is verbalised, whether in spoken or written form, the distress associated with it is reduced.

NAME IT 'I'm sad', 'I'm angry'. **OBSERVE IT** from the outside looking in. **NOTICE** how it is affecting your behaviour. Are you crying? Talking quickly? Clenching your fists? **TAKE A BREATH** and tell yourself it won't last forever. This is the hard bit! But like a broken bone, you will heal. You might be feeling sad or angry today, but tomorrow you will most likely feel different.

Now ask yourself where has this emotion come from? Don't blame yourself or anyone else for the emotion, just try to trace it back to its origin. Accept it and remind yourself it will pass.

USE THE TIPS ON PAGE 36 TO HELP YOU FLIP NEGATIVES INTO POSITIVES.

*Research by Katharina Kircanski, University of California (2012)

WHAT STRESSES ME OUT?

List some things that make you feel angry, sad, upset, anxious.

WHAT CAN I DO TO HELP REDUCE THE STRESS?

**** IF YOU ARE EXPERIENCING AN EXTENDED PERIOD OF SADNESS OR ANXIETY,
PLEASE TALK TO SOMEONE YOU TRUST OR A PROFESSIONAL ****

There are many different ways you can help manage negative emotions, so they don't linger.

FLIP THE NEGATIVE TO A POSITIVE

Instead of trying to calm yourself down by saying things like: "I am not anxious" try saying "I am excited!" Scientists have a simple, but radical, idea* that because both anxiety and excitement quicken your heartbeat, and put you in a state of high emotion, it is a shorter jump from anxious to excited, than from anxious to calm. So instead of fighting against your emotions, go with them, and embrace them. Change your focus from what could go wrong to what could go right. Focus on the good!

IDEAS FOR FLIPPING NEGATIVE ENERGY

EXERCISE – when you exercise your body releases some great chemicals that help you feel great, like dopamine. It is a great way to de-stress.

DO SOMETHING KIND FOR SOMEONE ELSE – this will help you to stop worrying about you, and focus on someone else.

TALK TO SOMEONE – telling people how you feel can make you feel better. If you feel sad but are not sure why, you could simply say that.

GET INTO NATURE – go for a walk on the beach, or in the bush. You don't need to talk, just surround yourself in the beauty of nature.

GRATITUDE – Of course! Write in this journal when you are feeling upset and try and flip your negative thoughts into positive ones. It can be hard at first but you will get better at it the more you practice. Think about all the things that are wonderful in your life. For tips on how to get the most outof your gratitude practice go to page twelve.

DISTRACTION – Try to do something else to take your mind off things. Try some mindfulness exercises like colouring in (page 125 and 172) or meditation, or put on your favourite music and dance around the room.

BREATHING – As mentioned in MANAGING EMOTIONS try diaphragmatic breathing to calm yourself down, you will find out how on page 122.

*Research by Alison Wood Brooks, Harvard Business School (2014)

CHALLENGING NEGATIVITY

By learning to use your rational 'resonable mind' responses while you are in an emotional state, you can take the sting out of negative thinking and the challenges that knock you down. Bringing attention to your thinking around your failures, and mistakes can help you to understand and accept them. You can learn to get back up again, keep going, and pursue your goals.

The 'reasonable mind' is driven by logic, the 'emotional mind' is driven by feelings, and the 'wise mind' is the middle-ground between the two. When you use diaphagmatic or deep belly breathing (see page 122) it helps you to STOP & THINK and your 'reasonable mind' kicks in before you react. If you are in an emotional state it is hard to make the best decision, and you might react badly to a situation. The same is also true if you were to use only the rational or logical side of our brain. By slowing down, and learning how to combine the two you are able to really think about not only your feelings but also about others, and make the best WISE decision that you can.

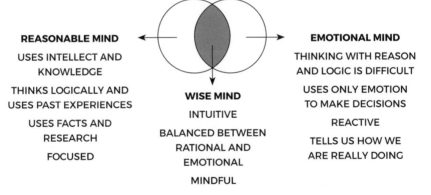

REASONABLE MIND

USES INTELLECT AND KNOWLEDGE

THINKS LOGICALLY AND USES PAST EXPERIENCES

USES FACTS AND RESEARCH

FOCUSED

WISE MIND

INTUITIVE

BALANCED BETWEEN RATIONAL AND EMOTIONAL

MINDFUL

EMOTIONAL MIND

THINKING WITH REASON AND LOGIC IS DIFFICULT

USES ONLY EMOTION TO MAKE DECISIONS

REACTIVE

TELLS US HOW WE ARE REALLY DOING

METHODS FOR FLIPPING NEGATIVE EMOTIONS

ANGER: Breathe deep and slow. Imagine breathing out the anger and breathing in calm. Do something that makes you happy. Use the list on page 14 for inspiration.

ANXIETY: Change your environment, use your breathing while you get out into nature. Track the origin of this emotion, and accept it.

GUILT: Remember we all make mistakes. Forgive yourself. Think about the times you have done something kind.

FEAR: Deep belly breaths. Imagine breathing out the fear and breathing in calm. Think about a time you have faced your fears in the past. Think about someone you admire. Do they have fears? Use your reasonable mind (see above).

Support can, and probably will, look different for everyone. The important thing to remember is that to really find that sense of belonging, the support, and connections in your life must be meaningful to you.

SOCIAL CONNECTION IS POWERFUL

Social connections can be found at home, at work, with friends, family, church, sports teams, volunteer groups, even online, anywhere you find people who provide you with meaning, and a sense of belonging. It's such an important part of our health and well-being that some governments, such as New Zealand, use social connectedness as one of its key indicators of the health of the country, and measure it regularly.

Good relationships keep us healthy and happier for longer. They keep us alive. In fact some studies* have found that social connection directly impacts how long you live, your immunity and ability to recover from disease, rates of depression and anxiety, self-esteem and empathy, emotional regulation. High social connectedness creates a positive feedback loop of social, emotional, and physical well-being.

It is not about the amount of friends you have, it is how meaningful your social connections are to you. JUST YOU. Do they give you a sense of purpose? Do they challenge you in a positive way to think differently, learn more? Do they make you feel safe and understood? Do they validate your values and contribution?

HOW TO BUILD SOCIAL CONNECTIONS

A sense of connection can be built by:

GIVING, SHARING, AND SUPPORTING OTHERS. This can be done through volunteering, joining a business network, mentoring others, or acts of kindness. There are prompts throughout this journal for acts of kindness or you can search online. There are plenty of ideas!

ASK FOR HELP. BE PROACTIVE. Take up invitations that you might assume are courtesy only. Find communities of practice that align with your values, goals, or aspirations. Join a social group like a book club, a sports team, a coffee group.

TAKING CARE OF YOURSELF. When we are stressed we tend to focus inwards. We stop thinking about, noticing, seeking, or responding to others. This starts a negative feedback loop and continues to decrease our connectivity. Use the tips to boost your mood on page 32 for ideas.

WHO OR WHAT IN MY SOCIAL NETWORK GIVES ME A SENSE OF PURPOSE AND IS MEANINGFUL?

e.g. family, friends, work, groups, organisations

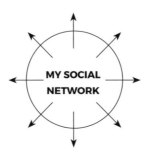

WHAT CAN I DO TO BUILD MY SENSE OF CONNECTION?

e.g. volunteering, participation, time management, join a group.

 USE THE HEALTHY HABIT TRACKER ON YOUR JOURNAL PAGES TO TRACK IF YOU MADE MEANINGFUL CONNECTIONS THAT DAY.

CONNECT

Find some time to read a book.

DATE

TODAY I AM GRATEFUL FOR...

HAPPINESS SCALE (%)

100

75

50

25

0

Thank You! Thank You! Thank You! Thank You! Thank You! Thank You!

HEALTHY HABITS

WORD FOR THE DAY

SLEEP   **MOVE**   **RELAX**   **CONNECT**

I
AM

POSITIVE AFFIRMATIONS

....

DATE

Good things are coming my way.

TODAY I AM GRATEFUL FOR...

HAPPINESS SCALE (%)

100

75

50

25

0

Thank You! Thank You! Thank You! Thank You! Thank You! Thank You!

HEALTHY HABITS

☹ 😐 ☺   ☹ 😐 ☺   ☹ 😐 ☺   ☹ 😐 ☺

SLEEP   **MOVE**   **RELAX**   **CONNECT**

WORD FOR THE DAY

POSITIVE AFFIRMATIONS

I AM

*Always trust your instinct, it will
lead you where you need to go.*

DATE

TODAY I AM GRATEFUL FOR...

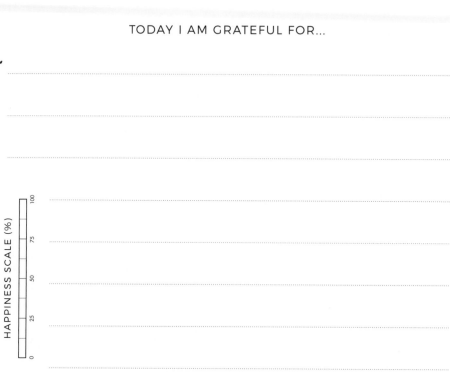

HAPPINESS SCALE (%)

100

75

50

25

0

Thank You! Thank You! Thank You! Thank You! Thank You! Thank You!

HEALTHY HABITS

SLEEP	MOVE	RELAX	CONNECT

WORD FOR THE DAY

I
AM

POSITIVE AFFIRMATIONS

Turn off your cell phone for the day.

DATE

WHAT WENT RIGHT THIS WEEK....

HAPPINESS SCALE (%)

100
75
50
25
0

Thank You! Thank You! Thank You! Thank You! Thank You! Thank You!

HEALTHY HABITS

SLEEP   **MOVE**   **RELAX**   **CONNECT**

WORD FOR THE DAY

MY STRENGTHS

Say "Good Morning" to a person standing next to you.

DATE

TODAY I AM GRATEFUL FOR...

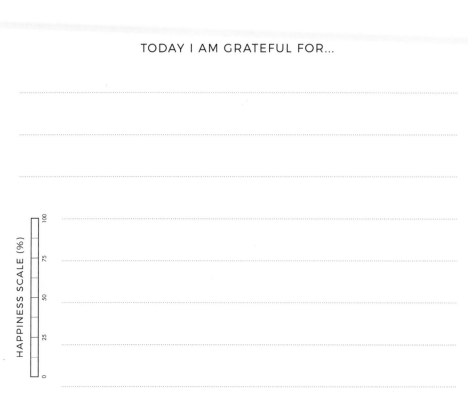

HAPPINESS SCALE (%)

100

75

50

25

0

Thank You! Thank You! Thank You! Thank You! Thank You! Thank You!

HEALTHY HABITS

WORD FOR THE DAY

SLEEP　　　**MOVE**　　　**RELAX**　　　**CONNECT**

I AM

POSITIVE AFFIRMATIONS

Pay attention to your thoughts,
they will become your future.

DATE

TODAY I AM GRATEFUL FOR...

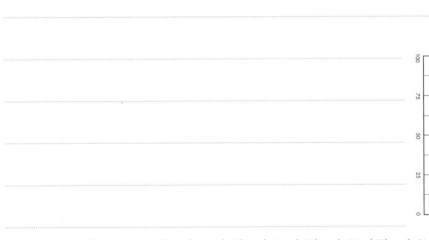

HAPPINESS SCALE (%)

100
75
50
25
0

Thank You! Thank You! Thank You! Thank You! Thank You! Thank You!

HEALTHY HABITS

SLEEP   **MOVE**   **RELAX**   **CONNECT**   WORD FOR THE DAY

POSITIVE AFFIRMATIONS

I
AM

Find something to believe in.

TODAY I AM GRATEFUL FOR...

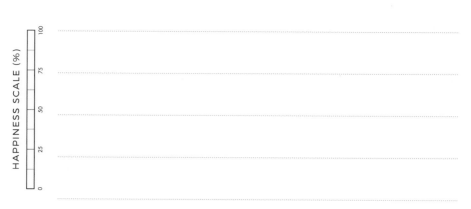

HAPPINESS SCALE (%)

100

75

50

25

0

Thank You! Thank You! Thank You! Thank You! Thank You! Thank You!

HEALTHY HABITS

WORD FOR THE DAY

SLEEP   **MOVE**   **RELAX**   **CONNECT**

I AM

POSITIVE AFFIRMATIONS

DATE

Today is a new day, a new
chance that I am so grateful for.

TODAY I AM GRATEFUL FOR...

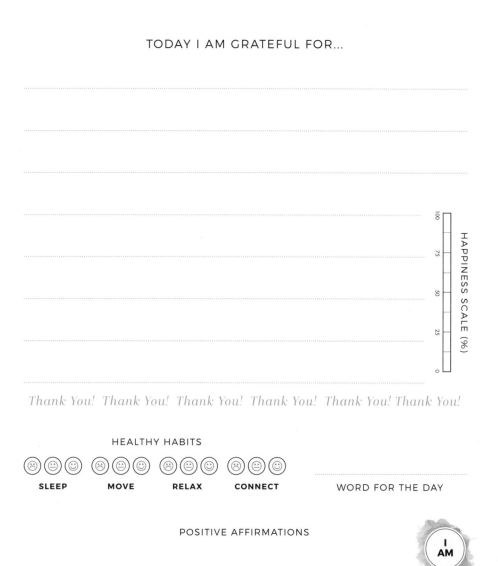

HAPPINESS SCALE (%)

100

75

50

25

0

Thank You! Thank You! Thank You! Thank You! Thank You! Thank You!

HEALTHY HABITS

SLEEP   **MOVE**   **RELAX**   **CONNECT**

WORD FOR THE DAY

POSITIVE AFFIRMATIONS

I AM

*Smile at as many people
as possible today.*

....

DATE

WHAT WENT RIGHT THIS WEEK....

....

....

....

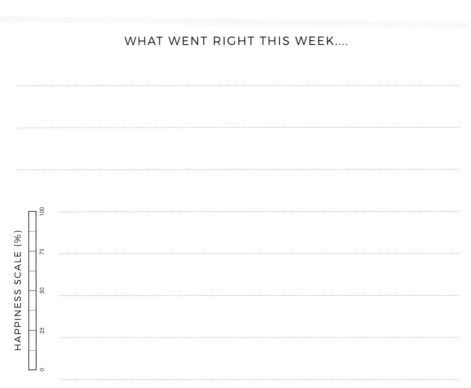

HAPPINESS SCALE (%)

100

75

50

25

0

Thank You! Thank You! Thank You! Thank You! Thank You! Thank You!

HEALTHY HABITS

SLEEP **MOVE** **RELAX** **CONNECT**

....

WORD FOR THE DAY

MY STRENGTHS

....

....

Today is the only day that
matters, what will you do with it?

DATE

TODAY I AM GRATEFUL FOR...

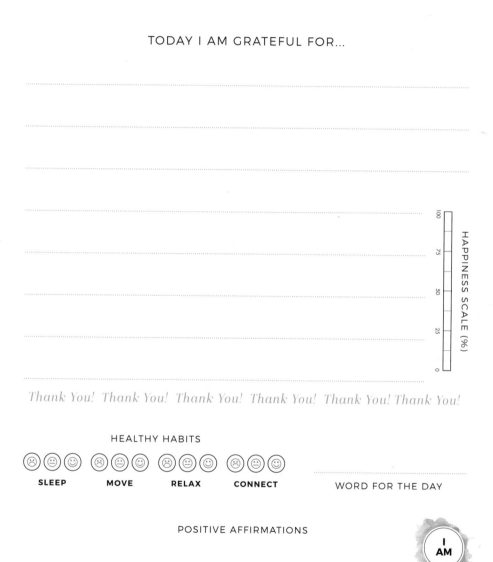

HAPPINESS SCALE (%)

100

75

50

25

0

Thank You! Thank You! Thank You! Thank You! Thank You! Thank You!

HEALTHY HABITS

SLEEP   **MOVE**   **RELAX**   **CONNECT**

WORD FOR THE DAY

POSITIVE AFFIRMATIONS

I
AM

Focus on changing the way you think and watch everything else change too.

DATE

TODAY I AM GRATEFUL FOR...

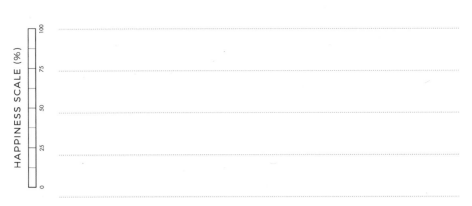

HAPPINESS SCALE (%)

100

75

50

25

0

Thank You! Thank You! Thank You! Thank You! Thank You! Thank You!

HEALTHY HABITS

| SLEEP | MOVE | RELAX | CONNECT |

WORD FOR THE DAY

I AM

POSITIVE AFFIRMATIONS

INSPIRATION

What are you waiting for?
You are the only one with
power over your world.

TODAY I AM GRATEFUL FOR...

HAPPINESS SCALE (%)

100

75

50

25

0

Thank You! Thank You! Thank You! Thank You! Thank You! Thank You!

HEALTHY HABITS

SLEEP   **MOVE**   **RELAX**   **CONNECT**

WORD FOR THE DAY

POSITIVE AFFIRMATIONS

I AM

Don't focus on your problems, let
your dreams show you the way.

DATE

TODAY I AM GRATEFUL FOR...

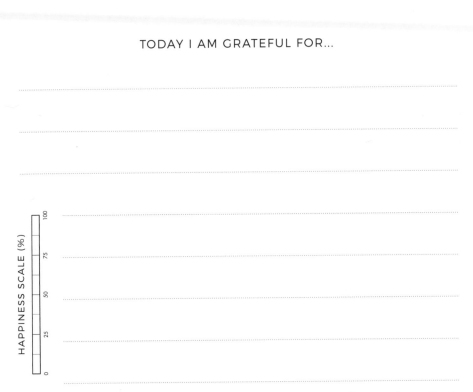

HAPPINESS SCALE (%)

100

75

50

25

0

Thank You! Thank You! Thank You! Thank You! Thank You! Thank You!

HEALTHY HABITS

SLEEP   **MOVE**   **RELAX**   **CONNECT**

WORD FOR THE DAY

I
AM

POSITIVE AFFIRMATIONS

WHAT WENT RIGHT THIS WEEK....

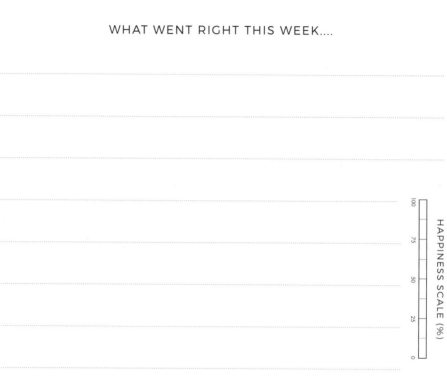

HAPPINESS SCALE (%)

100

75

50

25

0

Thank You! Thank You! Thank You! Thank You! Thank You! Thank You!

HEALTHY HABITS

SLEEP   **MOVE**   **RELAX**   **CONNECT**

WORD FOR THE DAY

MY STRENGTHS

Life is wonderful in its simplicity.

TODAY I AM GRATEFUL FOR...

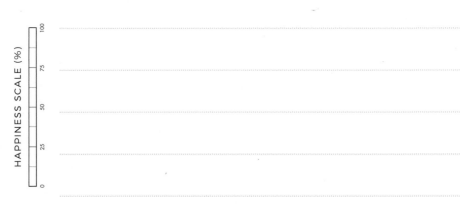

HAPPINESS SCALE (%)

100

75

50

25

0

Thank You! Thank You! Thank You! Thank You! Thank You! Thank You!

HEALTHY HABITS

WORD FOR THE DAY

SLEEP   **MOVE**   **RELAX**   **CONNECT**

I AM

POSITIVE AFFIRMATIONS

TODAY I AM GRATEFUL FOR...

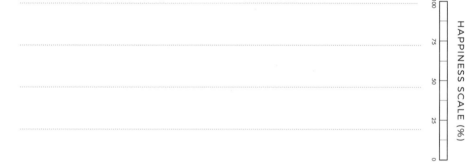

HAPPINESS SCALE (%)

100

75

50

25

0

Thank You! Thank You! Thank You! Thank You! Thank You! Thank You!

HEALTHY HABITS

SLEEP   **MOVE**   **RELAX**   **CONNECT**

WORD FOR THE DAY

POSITIVE AFFIRMATIONS

I AM

55

Write a love letter to yourself.

DATE

TODAY I AM GRATEFUL FOR...

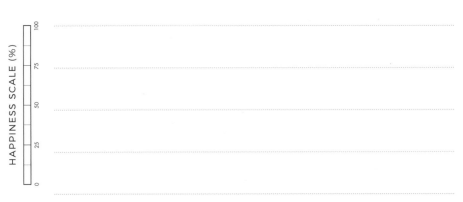

HAPPINESS SCALE (%)

100

75

50

25

0

Thank You! Thank You! Thank You! Thank You! Thank You! Thank You!

HEALTHY HABITS

SLEEP **MOVE** **RELAX** **CONNECT**

WORD FOR THE DAY

I
AM

POSITIVE AFFIRMATIONS

FOCUS ON
THE GOOD.
SOON YOU WILL
SEE MORE,
ENJOY MORE,
APPRECIATE MORE.

inspiration

Ever wanted to learn or do something new but told yourself you are not smart enough, or good enough, or you won't be able to do it? So you don't even try, or you give up?

TURN OFF YOUR INNER CRITIC

Called a fixed mindset, this thought pattern is like your very own personal critic, always in your head, telling you that you may as well give up because it's never going to happen, or you will fail, or look stupid in front of others, always focused on your weaknesses and flaws. But it doesn't have to be this way. You can learn to quiet that inner critic by changing your mindset to focus on your strengths, and your positive qualities. A GROWTH MINDSET means you approach new and challenging tasks with the view that you just don't know how to do it YET, rather than you can't do it at all.

WHAT KIND OF MINDSET DO YOU HAVE NOW?

Think of a skill or area you would like to be good at. It could be a job, a sport, your fitness, starting a business. Be honest with yourself. Where would you rate your beliefs about each of these areas? Mark in your score below out of 1-10.

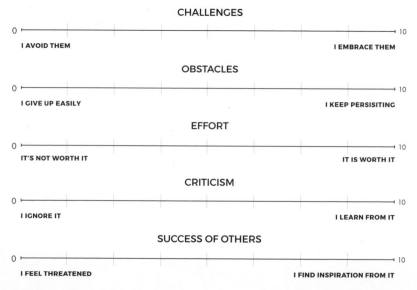

CHALLENGES

0 ⊢————————————————⊣ 10

I AVOID THEM   I EMBRACE THEM

OBSTACLES

0 ⊢————————————————⊣ 10

I GIVE UP EASILY   I KEEP PERSISITING

EFFORT

0 ⊢————————————————⊣ 10

IT'S NOT WORTH IT   IT IS WORTH IT

CRITICISM

0 ⊢————————————————⊣ 10

I IGNORE IT   I LEARN FROM IT

SUCCESS OF OTHERS

0 ⊢————————————————⊣ 10

I FEEL THREATENED   I FIND INSPIRATION FROM IT

LEARN TO FOSTER A GROWTH MINDSET AND FACE CHALLENGES WITHOUT FEAR

By believing your talents can be developed through hard work, perserverence, and good strategies you will be able to achieve more and be more motivated. By changing your focus you will put more energy into learning, and it will help you to feel empowered and committed.

It is easy to fall into defence mode or feel insecure when we receive criticism or face challenges, but this is a response that inhibits growth.

It is critical to reward yourself, not just for the effort you put in, but also for the process, progress and learning that helps you get there. Change the perspective of seeing mistakes as failure to a learning opportunity. Learn to capitalise on setbacks and challenging situations by learning new strategies and moving forward. You can develop, and grow your abilities to achieve your own personal goals.

First, and most importantly, recognise that it is possible, then think about the beliefs held by those with a growth mindset and ask yourself: Can I keep going? Where can I do better? What feedback have I been given, both positive and negative? Who already does this well? What can I learn from them?
Use the space at the back of this journal to work through these questions.

CHANGE YOUR MINDSET

Here are some examples of negative self-talk, from a fixed mindset perspective, and sentences to try instead. Use them as a guide and practice changing and reframing your words in your head.

INSTEAD OF THIS:	TRY THINKING THIS:
"I'm not good at this"	"What am I missing?"
"I may as well give up!"	"I'll use some of the things I have learned to keep trying."
"This is too hard!"	"This may take some time and effort."
"I never get things right!"	"I can always improve. I will keep trying."
"I made a mistake."	"Mistakes help me to learn."
"I'm a failure!"	"If I practice I will get better."
"I'll never be as successful as him/her."	"I'm going to figure out what he/she does and see if it works for me."
"This is as good as it will ever get."	"Is this really the best I can do?"

USE THE SPACE FOR WRITING ABOUT YOUR STRENGTHS ON YOUR JOURNAL PAGES TO CONCENTRATE ON WHAT YOU KNOW YOU CAN DO, OR WOULD LIKE TO DO.

Your mindset influences future thinking, behaviour, and how you make decisions. By focusing on your strengths, rather than your flaws, you can be more resourceful and resilient in the face of adversity.

STRENGTH-BASED APPROACH

In the same way that focusing on the good things in your life helps you to see more of the good and less of the hassles, so too is it true for the strength-based approach. By enhancing your strengths, and building on those characteristics that are present in you, you will begin to focus on them more than what you are not good at. You will more easily adapt and use those strengths in times of need.

THE SIMPLE TRICK IS TO FOCUS ON YOUR SKILLS, INTERESTS AND SUPPORT SYSTEMS. TO IDENTIFY WHAT IS GOING WELL, TO DO MORE OF IT, AND TO BUILD ON IT.

Your strengths don't mean how how fast you can run, or how much you know about technology. It means character strengths (e.g. honesty, positivity, persistence), personal strengths (e.g. imagination, focus, resilience), interpersonal strengths (e.g. persuasion, explaining, empathy), and organisational strengths (e.g. planning, problem solving, creating strategy). You need to figure out what comes naturally to you, that not everyone will find easy. What energises and motivates you?

POSITIVE WORDS I WOULD USE TO DESCRIBE MYSELF?

....

....

....

....

WHAT ARE MY UNIQUE ABILITIES?

WHAT CHALLENGES HAVE I OVERCOME?

WHAT DO OTHERS SAY I AM GOOD AT?

** FOCUSING YOUR ATTENTION INWARD AND LISTING YOUR STRENGTHS CAN MAKE YOU MORE
SELF-AWARE AND HELP YOU TO SEE WHERE YOU CAN IMPROVE. IF YOU NEED MORE ROOM, USE THE
SPACE AT THE BACK OF THIS JOURNAL TO NARROW DOWN WHAT IS MOST IMPORTANT TO YOU **

When your life choices don't match your values and beliefs you end up feeling dissatisfied, restless, angry, anxious and at worst unhappy.

WHAT IS YOUR WHY?

When you get your life choices right, for example what you do for a job, or in your spare time, the friends you spend time with — when they match your own values — you will feel satisfied, content, and at best energised and straight-up happy!

HOW TO FIND YOUR PURPOSE IN LIFE

Why is it that some people seem to be more successful when you have the same access to resources, education, or same amount of time in the day? Simon Sinek is a researcher who discovered a pattern to explain how. He suggests that the world's greatest leaders and innovators think, act and communicate in a way to drive consistent behaviour and thoughts that make them much more likely to succeed.

Everybody knows WHAT they do, some know HOW they do it, but very few people know WHY they do it. The very successful people or businesses KNOW their WHY, they know their passion and why they do what they do. The way the brain works drives their motivation, because their WHY is linked to their emotions and behaviours, whereas the WHAT is linked to rational thinking. By tuning into your WHY, you are motivated by a cause, a purpose, a belief that fuels your passion. If all you are motivated by is a result that is not fueled by emotion — more money, more followers, to be famous, to lose weight — then you are unlikely to succeed or be happy doing it.

WHAT DO YOU DO?

Relating to your job this could be, for example, are you in finance, hospitality, teaching? Do you look after a busy family, etc.?

HOW DO YOU DO IT?

How do you do that work, for example, full-time, part-time, solo, in a team, at home, in the office, in an executive environment, in a casual environment, in a traditional environment, in a progressive tech environment, commercially driven etc – whatever stands out as important to you.

WHY DO YOU DO IT?

What is the reasoning, passion or necessity behind why you do it, for example, innovation, to help others, creating something, being outdoors, stability, providing a future for your family – there really is no right or wrong here!

** IF YOU FIND THIS HARD USE THE SAME MODEL TO THINK ABOUT TIMES IN YOUR PAST WHEN YOU KNOW THAT YOU'VE FELT A SENSE OF SATISFACTION, CONTENTMENT AND ENERGY. WHAT ARE YOUR THEMES? DOES THE EXERCISE CHANGE THE WAY YOU THINK ABOUT YOUR JOB, YOUR FUTURE? WHAT WILL YOU DO ABOUT IT? **

Creating a vision board is another powerful tool to help align you with your deepest desires, and motivate you to reach your dream goals.

DEFINE WHAT YOU REALLY WANT IN YOUR LIFE.

If you don't know your why yet use this page to search deeply for the things that will really light up your life, for all you have ever dreamed of. What does your soul feel will empower you to be who you really are? What are your passions and your purpose?

MAKE AFFIRMATIONS ABOUT WHAT YOU WANT TO BE...

Making affirmations or positive statements, that describe your desired situation or goal, impress them on the subconscious mind. They serve to motivate, inspire and program your mind to act. e.g. I am successful; I am confident; I am a leading expert in interior design...

MAKE STATEMENTS ABOUT WHAT YOU WANT TO HAVE...

What do you desire? e.g. A beach house, a new car, true love, health or wealth? Be specific.

MAKE STATEMENTS ABOUT WHAT YOU WANT TO DO...

If money were no object what would you do? e.g. Travel to inspiring places, help others, build a business...

....

....

....

....

ASK FOR IT. BELIEVE IT. RECEIVE IT.

MY WISH LIST...

If you could manifest ANYTHING what would be your TOP 10?

1. ....   6. ....

2. ....   7. ....

3. ....   8. ....

4. ....   9. ....

5. ....   10. ....

Use the words from this page for inspiration to create a Life Map/vision board, and put it somewhere you will see and notice it everyday. The more often you see and read your goals, the more results you will get. Review and revise your goals regularly. Try experimenting with different ways of stating your goals. Stay positive and set goals over which you have as much control as possible, your own personal performance and attitude.

**VISION BOARD STARTER PACKS ARE AVAILABLE FROM AWESOME INC.
WWW.THEAWESOMEINC.CO.NZ**

*The more grateful you become
the easier it is to be grateful.*

DATE

TODAY I AM GRATEFUL FOR...

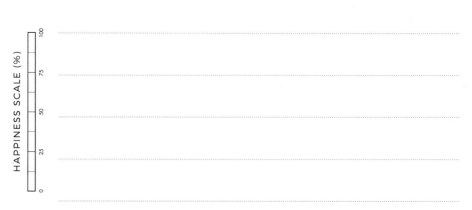

HAPPINESS SCALE (%)

100

75

50

25

0

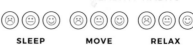

Thank You! Thank You! Thank You! Thank You! Thank You! Thank You!

HEALTHY HABITS

WORD FOR THE DAY

SLEEP   **MOVE**   **RELAX**   **CONNECT**

I
AM

POSITIVE AFFIRMATIONS

*We are creatures of habit, so make
sure your habits are good ones.*

WHAT WENT RIGHT THIS WEEK....

HAPPINESS SCALE (%)

100

75

50

25

0

Thank You! Thank You! Thank You! Thank You! Thank You! Thank You!

HEALTHY HABITS

SLEEP   **MOVE**   **RELAX**   **CONNECT**

WORD FOR THE DAY

MY STRENGTHS

I am excited about the future.

DATE

TODODAY I AM GRATEFUL FOR...

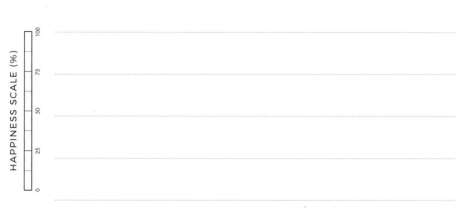

HAPPINESS SCALE (%)

100

75

50

25

0

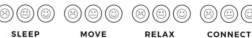

Thank You! Thank You! Thank You! Thank You! Thank You! Thank You!

HEALTHY HABITS

WORD FOR THE DAY

SLEEP   **MOVE**   **RELAX**   **CONNECT**

I
AM

POSITIVE AFFIRMATIONS

Reconnect with someone
you haven't seen in a while.

DATE

TODAY I AM GRATEFUL FOR...

HAPPINESS SCALE (%)

100

75

50

25

0

Thank You! Thank You! Thank You! Thank You! Thank You! Thank You!

HEALTHY HABITS

SLEEP   **MOVE**   **RELAX**   **CONNECT**

WORD FOR THE DAY

POSITIVE AFFIRMATIONS

I AM

Think about what you truly
love and invest time in it.

DATE

TODAY I AM GRATEFUL FOR...

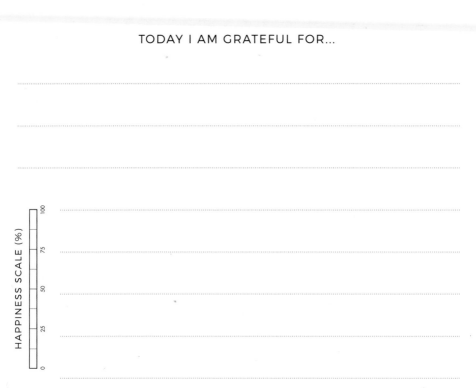

HAPPINESS SCALE (%)

100

75

50

25

0

Thank You! Thank You! Thank You! Thank You! Thank You! Thank You!

HEALTHY HABITS

WORD FOR THE DAY

SLEEP **MOVE** **RELAX** **CONNECT**

I
AM

POSITIVE AFFIRMATIONS

Get out into the garden today, do some weeding or plant some vegetables.

DATE

TODAY I AM GRATEFUL FOR...

HAPPINESS SCALE (%)

100

75

50

25

0

Thank You! Thank You! Thank You! Thank You! Thank You! Thank You!

HEALTHY HABITS

SLEEP   **MOVE**   **RELAX**   **CONNECT**

WORD FOR THE DAY

POSITIVE AFFIRMATIONS

I AM

71

Buy yourself a new piece of clothing.

DATE

WHAT WENT RIGHT THIS WEEK....

HAPPINESS SCALE (%)

100

75

50

25

0

Thank You! Thank You! Thank You! Thank You! Thank You! Thank You!

HEALTHY HABITS

SLEEP   **MOVE**   **RELAX**   **CONNECT**

WORD FOR THE DAY

MY STRENGTHS

DATE

Sometimes things not falling into place can be the luckiest thing that ever happened.

TODAY I AM GRATEFUL FOR...

HAPPINESS SCALE (%)

100

75

50

25

0

Thank You! Thank You! Thank You! Thank You! Thank You! Thank You!

HEALTHY HABITS

SLEEP   **MOVE**   **RELAX**   **CONNECT**

WORD FOR THE DAY

POSITIVE AFFIRMATIONS

I AM

Dance.

DATE

TODAY I AM GRATEFUL FOR...

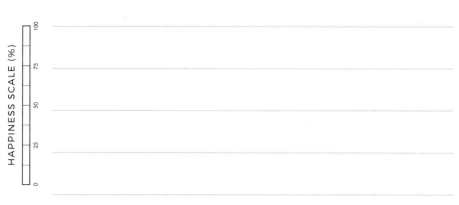

HAPPINESS SCALE (%)

100

75

50

25

0

Thank You! Thank You! Thank You! Thank You! Thank You! Thank You!

HEALTHY HABITS

WORD FOR THE DAY

SLEEP　　**MOVE**　　**RELAX**　　**CONNECT**

I AM

POSITIVE AFFIRMATIONS

Believe in yourself!

....
DATE

TODAY I AM GRATEFUL FOR...

HAPPINESS SCALE (%)

100
75
50
25
0

Thank You! Thank You! Thank You! Thank You! Thank You! Thank You!

HEALTHY HABITS

SLEEP   **MOVE**   **RELAX**   **CONNECT**

WORD FOR THE DAY

POSITIVE AFFIRMATIONS

I AM

Dance some more.

DATE

TODAY I AM GRATEFUL FOR...

HAPPINESS SCALE (%)

100

75

50

25

0

Thank You! Thank You! Thank You! Thank You! Thank You! Thank You!

HEALTHY HABITS

WORD FOR THE DAY

SLEEP   **MOVE**   **RELAX**   **CONNECT**

I
AM

POSITIVE AFFIRMATIONS

....

DATE

I am calm and rested, ready for the day.

WHAT WENT RIGHT THIS WEEK....

....

....

....

....

....

....

....

HAPPINESS SCALE (%)

100
75
50
25
0

....

Thank You! Thank You! Thank You! Thank You! Thank You! Thank You!

HEALTHY HABITS

SLEEP   **MOVE**   **RELAX**   **CONNECT**

WORD FOR THE DAY

MY STRENGTHS

....

....

Be open for opportunities that
come your way and take a chance
on them.

DATE

TODAY I AM GRATEFUL FOR...

HAPPINESS SCALE (%)

100

75

50

25

0

Thank You! Thank You! Thank You! Thank You! Thank You! Thank You!

HEALTHY HABITS

WORD FOR THE DAY   **SLEEP**   **MOVE**   **RELAX**   **CONNECT**

I
AM

POSITIVE AFFIRMATIONS

Kiss someone you love.

DATE

TODAY I AM GRATEFUL FOR...

HAPPINESS SCALE (%)

100

75

50

25

0

Thank You! Thank You! Thank You! Thank You! Thank You! Thank You!

HEALTHY HABITS

SLEEP   MOVE   RELAX   CONNECT

WORD FOR THE DAY

POSITIVE AFFIRMATIONS

I AM

Expect nothing,
appreciate everything.

THANKING OTHERS

Say 'thank you' as often as you can to as many people as you can.

Thank them for the little things, like holding a lift door for you, but also for the big stuff too, like your parents for their support growing up.

Simply saying 'thank you' to a spouse can create a virtuous cycle of gratitude, where each person feels more appreciated and happy.

Not only will it make them feel happy but it will make you feel more positive emotions, relish good experiences, improve your health, plus help you deal with adversity and build stronger relationships.*

The positive action of thanking someone directly for what they have done for YOU can also contribute to that person's feelings for you—they see you as kinder, more loving, and even more attractive.**

*Emmons, R., and Stern, R. (2013) Gratitude as a Psychotherapeutic Intervention. *Journal of Clinical Psychology*, Vol. 69(8), 846-855
**Algoe, S.B; Kurtz, L.E., & Hilaire, N.M. (2016) Putting the "you" in "thank you": Examining other-praising behavior as the active relational ingredient in expressed gratitude. *Social Psychological and Personality Science*, Vol. 7(7) 658-666

IF YOU CAN IMAGINE IT, IT IS YOURS FOR THE TAKING.

inspiration

If your brain is not getting the right nutrients to function at its best, you may be left feeling anxious, sad or uneasy.

FEED YOUR MIND

Crowding in foods that support your brain, as well as engaging in certain lifestyle changes, can potentially enhance how you're feeling overall, both mentally and physically. If the brain is not getting the nutrients it needs, this can manifest into symptoms of anxiety and sadness, as well as other feelings of general unease.

NOURISH YOUR BODY AND MIND
WITH HEALTHY REAL FOOD

If all you do is eat food that has gone through the least amount of processing possible, you're off to a great start, as you're naturally reducing those foods that can contribute to feeling poorly, and increasing food that is nutrient dense. Experiment with different vegetables, whole grains, proteins, fats and carbs and take note of how you feel after you eat. Are you feeling sluggish, bloated, anxious, sleepy?

If certain foods make you feel uncomfortable or irritable, you don't need to starve yourself or diet, just listen to your body and crowd in the foods that make you feel amazing, and adjust what you eat accordingly.

When it comes to mood, we can't neglect the role our gut plays. Serotonin the 'happy making' transmitter is formulated in the gut, not the brain, so we need to keep it happy. Research* is emerging showing a strong link between gut bacteria and our mind. The good bacteria secrete a massive amount of chemicals and in these chemicals are the same substances used to communicate and regulate mood. Chemicals like dopamine, serotonin, and gamma-aminobutyric acid (GABA), all of which affect feelings of anxiety, and depression.

Try incorporating some foods that give your gut some love like: probiotic foods, fatty fish, fibre, resistent starches, foods that reduce inflammation like tumeric, and lots of vegetables and fruit.

Remember a little bit of processed food that you love and enjoy here and there won't affect your mental health. if you truly enjoy it, guilt free, and in moderation.

READ MORE ABOUT CROWDING IN AND GENTLE NUTRITION AT
WWW.THEAWESOMEINC.CO.NZ/BLOGS/NUTRITION

*Research by Megan Clapp et al, Texas Tech University, USA (201"
& Jane A. Foster, McMaster University, Ontario, Canada (201.

FOOD THAT HAS AN EFFECT ON ME

Make a list of foods you have noticed make your body feel uncomfortable,
sluggish, bloated, anxious, or sleepy. Try to avoid these foods.

....

....

....

....

....

....

FOOD THAT MAKES ME FEEL AMAZING

Make a list of foods that give you energy, clarity and focus.
Crowd in these foods!

....

....

....

....

....

....

Focus on the good,
eat real food, move often, sleep well...
Feel amazing!

Sleep is very important for helping you to function at your best, both physically AND mentally.

CREATE HEALTHY SLEEP HABITS

Getting enough sleep is essential to your well-being, and skipping sleep, or not getting enough, can make you feel moody and irritable. Lack of sleep can stop you performing at your best, whether playing sport or performing at work. It limits your ability to concentrate or problem solve and can even make you more aggressive or make you more prone to getting sick.

Adults require seven to nine hours sleep a night, but sometimes you may think you can get by on less, or you have bedtime habits that contribute to poor sleep. Make sure to pay attention to your mood, energy and health after a bad night's sleep compared to a good one.

HOW TO GET ENOUGH GOOD QUALITY SLEEP

1. Your bedroom should be your sanctuary, keep it cool, dark and as quiet as possible. Make sure your bed, mattress and pillow are comfortable and inviting.
2. Exercise daily, even if just a gentle walk. See more information on pages 152-155.
3. Don't drink alcohol, caffeine, energy, or high sugar drinks before bed. In particular alcohol can have a significant effect on your recovery during sleep.
4. Keep your smart phone, TV and other devices out of the bedroom, or turn them off an hour before bed.
5. Establish a regular bed-time ritual that helps you to relax and wind down — brush your teeth, create a pampering ritual, and write in this journal, or read a book — your body will soon learn the signals for when it is time to go to sleep.
6. Aim to go to sleep and wake up at the same time every day.*

USE THE HEALTHY HABIT TRACKER ON YOUR JOURNAL PAGES TO TRACK YOUR SLEEP. WAS IT BAD, OK OR GOOD? CHECK FOR PATTERNS AND SEE IF SLEEP AFFECTS YOUR MOOD, OR IS RELATED TO OTHER HABITS.

SLEEP

*Tips www.sleepfoundation.org

....

DATE

*At any moment you can decide
to change your life. Choose now.*

TODAY I AM GRATEFUL FOR...

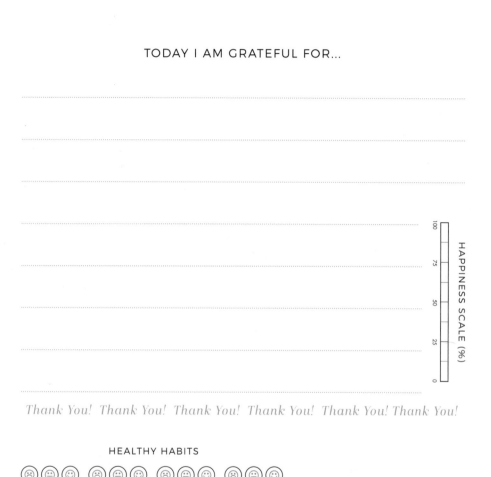

HAPPINESS SCALE (%)

100

75

50

25

0

Thank You! Thank You! Thank You! Thank You! Thank You! Thank You!

HEALTHY HABITS

| SLEEP | MOVE | RELAX | CONNECT |

WORD FOR THE DAY

POSITIVE AFFIRMATIONS

I AM

85

Do something different today from your usual routine.

DATE

TODAY I AM GRATEFUL FOR...

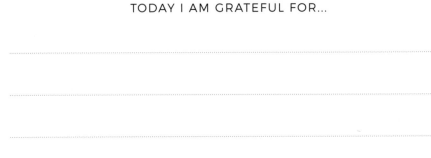

HAPPINESS SCALE (%)

100

75

50

25

0

Thank You! Thank You! Thank You! Thank You! Thank You! Thank You!

HEALTHY HABITS

WORD FOR THE DAY

SLEEP   **MOVE**   **RELAX**   **CONNECT**

I AM

POSITIVE AFFIRMATIONS

DATE

Don't focus on your problems, let
your dreams show you the way.

WHAT WENT RIGHT THIS WEEK....

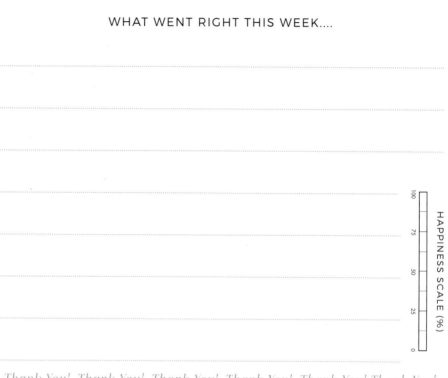

HAPPINESS SCALE (%)

100
75
50
25
0

Thank You! Thank You! Thank You! Thank You! Thank You! Thank You!

HEALTHY HABITS

SLEEP　　**MOVE**　　**RELAX**　　**CONNECT**

WORD FOR THE DAY

MY STRENGTHS

Write a letter of gratitude to someone
(you don't have to actually send it).

DATE

TODAY I AM GRATEFUL FOR...

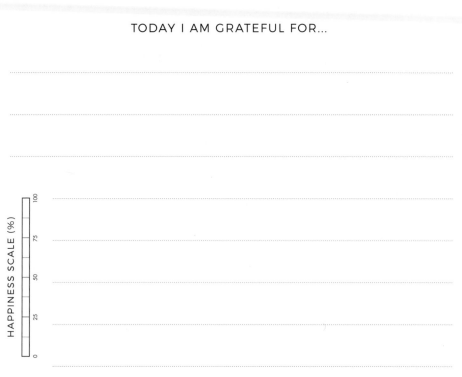

HAPPINESS SCALE (%)

100

75

50

25

0

Thank You! Thank You! Thank You! Thank You! Thank You! Thank You!

HEALTHY HABITS

SLEEP	MOVE	RELAX	CONNECT

WORD FOR THE DAY

I AM

POSITIVE AFFIRMATIONS

There are so many beautiful
reasons to be happy today.

DATE

TODAY I AM GRATEFUL FOR...

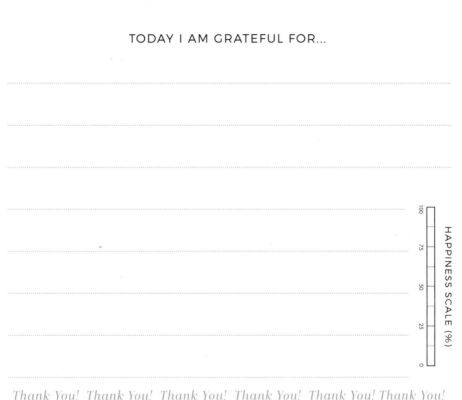

HAPPINESS SCALE (%)

Thank You! Thank You! Thank You! Thank You! Thank You! Thank You!

HEALTHY HABITS

SLEEP   **MOVE**   **RELAX**   **CONNECT**

WORD FOR THE DAY

POSITIVE AFFIRMATIONS

I AM

*It really is the simple things
in life that matter.*

························
DATE

TODAY I AM GRATEFUL FOR...

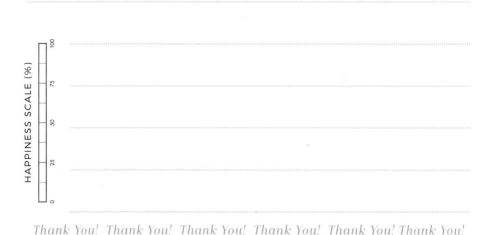

HAPPINESS SCALE (%)

100

75

50

25

0

Thank You! Thank You! Thank You! Thank You! Thank You! Thank You!

HEALTHY HABITS

WORD FOR THE DAY   **SLEEP**   **MOVE**   **RELAX**   **CONNECT**

I
AM

POSITIVE AFFIRMATIONS

The more you focus on the good things,
the better your life will become.

....
DATE

TODAY I AM GRATEFUL FOR...

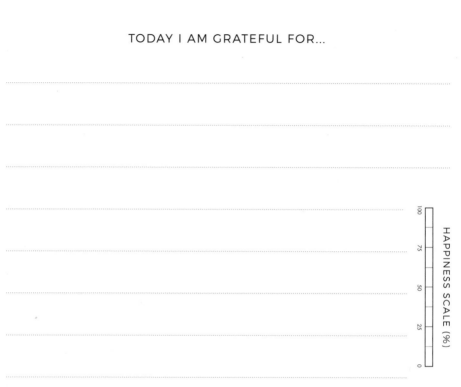

HAPPINESS SCALE (%)

100
75
50
25
0

Thank You! Thank You! Thank You! Thank You! Thank You! Thank You!

HEALTHY HABITS

SLEEP   **MOVE**   **RELAX**   **CONNECT**

WORD FOR THE DAY

POSITIVE AFFIRMATIONS

I AM

Today choose happiness at
every chance you get.

DATE

WHAT WENT RIGHT THIS WEEK....

HAPPINESS SCALE (%)

100

75

50

25

0

Thank You! Thank You! Thank You! Thank You! Thank You! Thank You!

HEALTHY HABITS

WORD FOR THE DAY

SLEEP   **MOVE**   **RELAX**   **CONNECT**

MY STRENGTHS

TODAY I AM GRATEFUL FOR...

HAPPINESS SCALE (%)

100

75

50

25

0

Thank You! Thank You! Thank You! Thank You! Thank You! Thank You!

HEALTHY HABITS

☹ 😐 ☺ ☹ 😐 ☺ ☹ 😐 ☺ ☹ 😐 ☺

SLEEP   **MOVE**   **RELAX**   **CONNECT**

WORD FOR THE DAY

POSITIVE AFFIRMATIONS

I AM

Do something adventurous.

DATE

TODAY I AM GRATEFUL FOR...

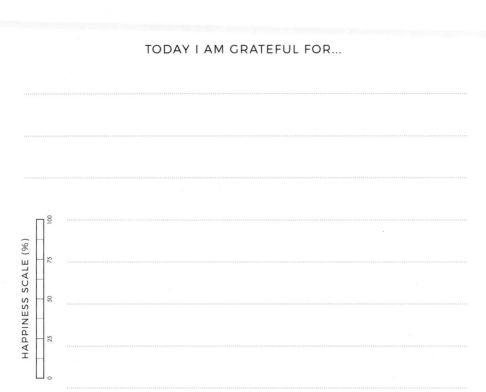

HAPPINESS SCALE (%)

100

75

50

25

0

Thank You! Thank You! Thank You! Thank You! Thank You! Thank You!

HEALTHY HABITS

WORD FOR THE DAY

SLEEP   **MOVE**   **RELAX**   **CONNECT**

I AM

POSITIVE AFFIRMATIONS

Buy a stranger lunch today.

....

DATE

TODAY I AM GRATEFUL FOR...

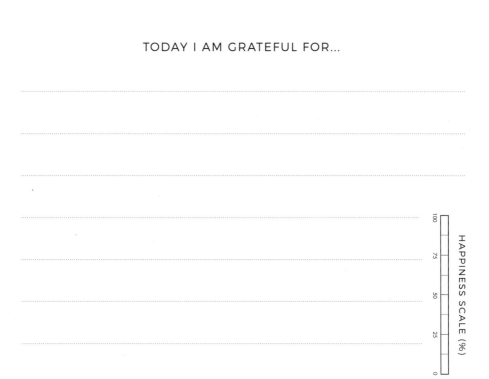

HAPPINESS SCALE (%)

100

75

50

25

0

Thank You! Thank You! Thank You! Thank You! Thank You! Thank You!

HEALTHY HABITS

SLEEP　　**MOVE**　　**RELAX**　　**CONNECT**

WORD FOR THE DAY

POSITIVE AFFIRMATIONS

I
AM

Stop what you are doing and breathe.

DATE

TODAY I AM GRATEFUL FOR...

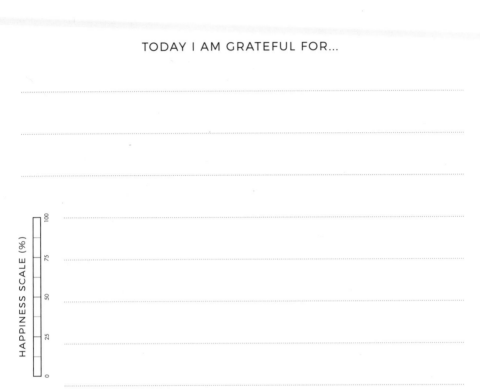

HAPPINESS SCALE (%)

100

75

50

25

0

Thank You! Thank You! Thank You! Thank You! Thank You! Thank You!

HEALTHY HABITS

WORD FOR THE DAY

SLEEP   **MOVE**   **RELAX**   **CONNECT**

I
AM

POSITIVE AFFIRMATIONS

Remember you have amazing
untapped potential inside you.

DATE
....

WHAT WENT RIGHT THIS WEEK....

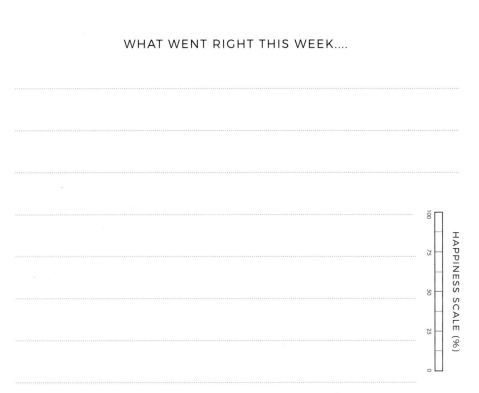

HAPPINESS SCALE (%)

100
75
50
25
0

Thank You! Thank You! Thank You! Thank You! Thank You! Thank You!

HEALTHY HABITS

SLEEP   **MOVE**   **RELAX**   **CONNECT**

WORD FOR THE DAY

MY STRENGTHS

Find time to fit in some stillness and quiet. Time to connect with your inner self.

DATE

TODAY I AM GRATEFUL FOR...

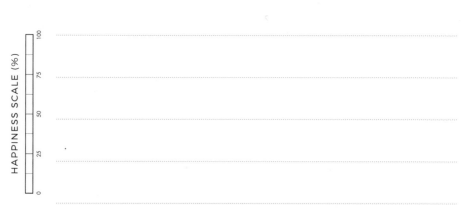

HAPPINESS SCALE (%)

100

75

50

25

0

Thank You! Thank You! Thank You! Thank You! Thank You! Thank You!

HEALTHY HABITS

WORD FOR THE DAY

 SLEEP   **MOVE**   **RELAX** **CONNECT**

 I AM

POSITIVE AFFIRMATIONS

TODAY I AM GRATEFUL FOR...

HAPPINESS SCALE (%)

100

75

50

25

0

Thank You! Thank You! Thank You! Thank You! Thank You! Thank You!

HEALTHY HABITS

SLEEP   **MOVE**   **RELAX**   **CONNECT**

WORD FOR THE DAY

POSITIVE AFFIRMATIONS

I
AM

*Happiness and
good vibes are contagious.
Help spread them.*

LAUGH A LOT

Laugh as much as you can, whenever you can, and learn to laugh at yourself too.

As the saying goes – laughter is the best medicine. Even if you force yourself to laugh, by faking it, for long enough, at some point you will genuinely start laughing. Research into the effects of laughter show it activates endorphins and other feel-good neurotransmitters in your brain, which aids in strengthening your immune system, help boosts your energy, and diminishes pain, and also protects you from the effects of stress.[*]

It can instantly lift your mood, which relaxes the body and often this feeling can stay with you long after the laughter subsides. One study found that incorporating bouts of simulated laughter into an exercise program helped improve older adults' mental health as well as their aerobic endurance.[**]

[*]Bennett, M. P., & Lengacher, C. (2008). Humor and laughter may influence health: III. Laughter and health outcomes. *Evidence-Based Complementary and Alternative Medicine* :eCAM, 5(1), 37–40.
[**]Greene, C. M., Morgan , J. C., Traywick, L. S., and Mingo, C. A. (2017) Evaluation of a laughter-based exercise program on health and self-efficacy for exercise. *The Gerontologist*, 57: 6, 1051–1061

Be fearless and light up your soul.

·····································
DATE

TODAY I AM GRATEFUL FOR...

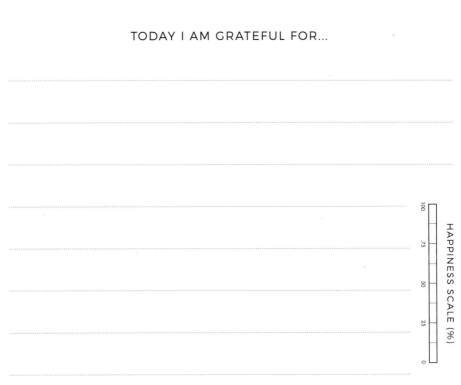

HAPPINESS SCALE (%)

100

75

50

25

0

Thank You! Thank You! Thank You! Thank You! Thank You! Thank You!

HEALTHY HABITS

SLEEP   **MOVE**   **RELAX**   **CONNECT**   WORD FOR THE DAY

POSITIVE AFFIRMATIONS

I AM

....

DATE

TODAY I AM GRATEFUL FOR...

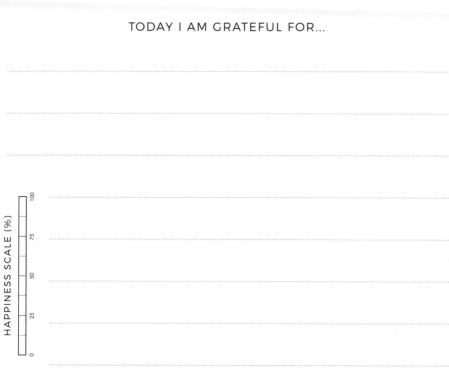

HAPPINESS SCALE (%)

100

75

50

25

0

Thank You! Thank You! Thank You! Thank You! Thank You! Thank You!

HEALTHY HABITS

WORD FOR THE DAY

SLEEP   **MOVE**   **RELAX**   **CONNECT**

I
AM

POSITIVE AFFIRMATIONS

Do someone a favour without asking for anything in return.

DATE

WHAT WENT RIGHT THIS WEEK....

HAPPINESS SCALE (%)

100

75

50

25

0

Thank You! Thank You! Thank You! Thank You! Thank You! Thank You!

HEALTHY HABITS

SLEEP   **MOVE**   **RELAX**   **CONNECT**

WORD FOR THE DAY

MY STRENGTHS

★

*Go outside and yell to
the Universe 'Thank You!'*

DATE

TODAY I AM GRATEFUL FOR...

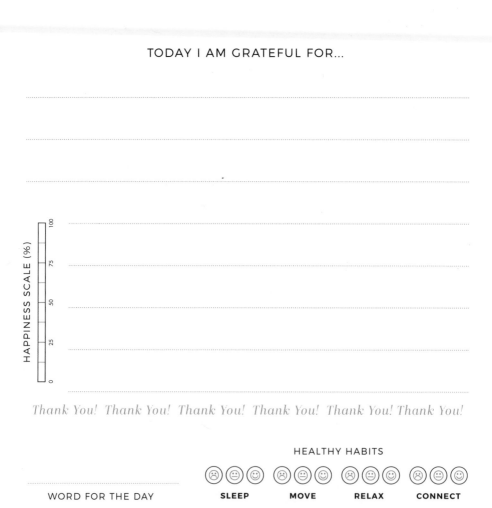

HAPPINESS SCALE (%)

100

75

50

25

0

Thank You! Thank You! Thank You! Thank You! Thank You! Thank You!

HEALTHY HABITS

| SLEEP | MOVE | RELAX | CONNECT |

WORD FOR THE DAY

I AM

POSITIVE AFFIRMATIONS

*Today is a good day to
change your life.*

....
DATE

TODAY I AM GRATEFUL FOR...

....

....

....

....

HAPPINESS SCALE (%)

100

75

50

25

0

....

....

....

Thank You! Thank You! Thank You! Thank You! Thank You! Thank You!

HEALTHY HABITS

SLEEP　　**MOVE**　　**RELAX**　　**CONNECT**

WORD FOR THE DAY

POSITIVE AFFIRMATIONS

I
AM

....

....

Say something kind to a stranger.

DATE

TODAY I AM GRATEFUL FOR...

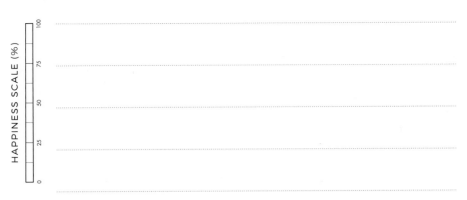

HAPPINESS SCALE (%)

100
75
50
25
0

Thank You! Thank You! Thank You! Thank You! Thank You! Thank You!

HEALTHY HABITS

WORD FOR THE DAY

SLEEP   MOVE   RELAX   CONNECT

I AM

POSITIVE AFFIRMATIONS

....

DATE

Do something fun! Go to a theme park or sign up for an adventure.

TODAY I AM GRATEFUL FOR...

....

....

....

....

....

....

....

HAPPINESS SCALE (%)

100

75

50

25

0

Thank You! Thank You! Thank You! Thank You! Thank You! Thank You!

HEALTHY HABITS

SLEEP   **MOVE**   **RELAX**   **CONNECT**

WORD FOR THE DAY

....

POSITIVE AFFIRMATIONS

I AM

....

....

Start your day with a positive thought.

DATE

WHAT WENT RIGHT THIS WEEK....

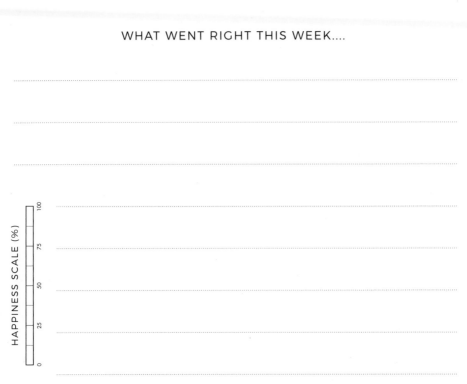

HAPPINESS SCALE (%)

100

75

50

25

0

Thank You! Thank You! Thank You! Thank You! Thank You! Thank You!

HEALTHY HABITS

WORD FOR THE DAY

SLEEP   **MOVE**   **RELAX**   **CONNECT**

MY STRENGTHS

DATE

When you stop being busy and look around, life really is astonishing.

TODAY I AM GRATEFUL FOR...

HAPPINESS SCALE (%)

100

75

50

25

0

Thank You! Thank You! Thank You! Thank You! Thank You! Thank You!

HEALTHY HABITS

SLEEP   **MOVE**   **RELAX**   **CONNECT**

WORD FOR THE DAY

POSITIVE AFFIRMATIONS

I AM

Tell someone they are beautiful today.

DATE

TODAY I AM GRATEFUL FOR...

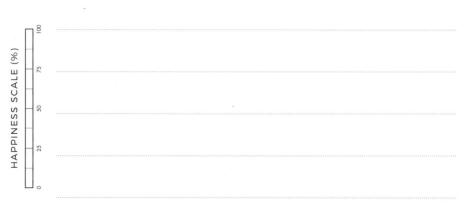

HAPPINESS SCALE (%)

100

75

50

25

0

Thank You! Thank You! Thank You! Thank You! Thank You! Thank You!

HEALTHY HABITS

SLEEP	MOVE	RELAX	CONNECT

WORD FOR THE DAY

I AM

POSITIVE AFFIRMATIONS

DATE

TODAY I AM GRATEFUL FOR...

HAPPINESS SCALE (%)

100

75

50

25

0

Thank You! Thank You! Thank You! Thank You! Thank You! Thank You!

HEALTHY HABITS

SLEEP　　**MOVE**　　**RELAX**　　**CONNECT**

WORD FOR THE DAY

POSITIVE AFFIRMATIONS

I AM

*Sign up to regularly
donate to a charity.*

DATE

TODAY I AM GRATEFUL FOR...

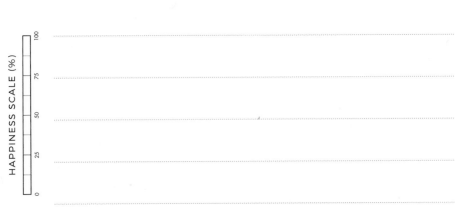

HAPPINESS SCALE (%)

100

75

50

25

0

Thank You! Thank You! Thank You! Thank You! Thank You! Thank You!

HEALTHY HABITS

SLEEP   MOVE   RELAX   CONNECT

WORD FOR THE DAY

I
AM

POSITIVE AFFIRMATIONS

Tear down the walls that keep
you locked in the sameness.

WHAT WENT RIGHT THIS WEEK....

HAPPINESS SCALE (%)

100

75

50

25

0

Thank You! Thank You! Thank You! Thank You! Thank You! Thank You!

HEALTHY HABITS

SLEEP   MOVE   RELAX   CONNECT

WORD FOR THE DAY

MY STRENGTHS

★

Something amazing could
happen today if you believe it.

DATE

TODAY I AM GRATEFUL FOR...

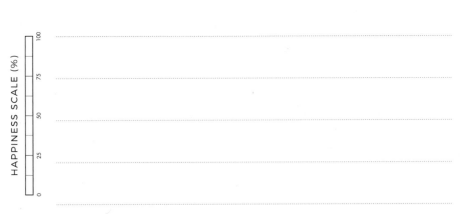

HAPPINESS SCALE (%)

100

75

50

25

0

Thank You! Thank You! Thank You! Thank You! Thank You! Thank You!

HEALTHY HABITS

WORD FOR THE DAY

SLEEP   **MOVE**   **RELAX**   **CONNECT**

I
AM

POSITIVE AFFIRMATIONS

DATE

....

TODAY I AM GRATEFUL FOR...

HAPPINESS SCALE (%)

100

75

50

25

0

Thank You! Thank You! Thank You! Thank You! Thank You! Thank You!

HEALTHY HABITS

☹ 😐 ☺   ☹ 😐 ☺   ☹ 😐 ☺   ☹ 😐 ☺

SLEEP   **MOVE**   **RELAX**   **CONNECT**

WORD FOR THE DAY

POSITIVE AFFIRMATIONS

I
AM

Choose to live, not to merely exist.

DATE

TODAY I AM GRATEFUL FOR...

HAPPINESS SCALE (%)

100

75

50

25

0

Thank You! Thank You! Thank You! Thank You! Thank You! Thank You!

HEALTHY HABITS

SLEEP   **MOVE**   **RELAX**   **CONNECT**

WORD FOR THE DAY

I
AM

POSITIVE AFFIRMATIONS

Happiness is simply a
by-product of gratitude.

DATE

TODAY I AM GRATEFUL FOR...

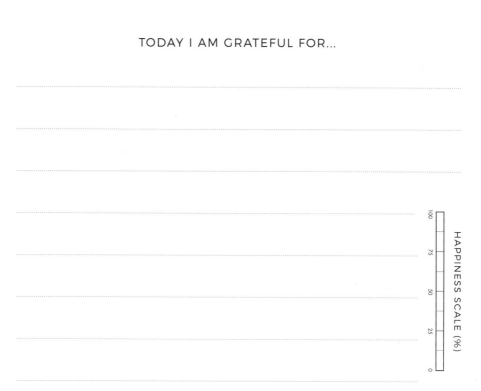

HAPPINESS SCALE (%)

100
75
50
25
0

Thank You! Thank You! Thank You! Thank You! Thank You! Thank You!

HEALTHY HABITS

SLEEP   **MOVE**   **RELAX**   **CONNECT**

WORD FOR THE DAY

POSITIVE AFFIRMATIONS

I
AM

Treat yourself to something you
have wanted for a long time.

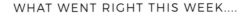

DATE

WHAT WENT RIGHT THIS WEEK....

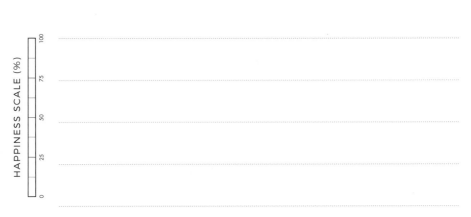

HAPPINESS SCALE (%)

100

75

50

25

0

Thank You! Thank You! Thank You! Thank You! Thank You! Thank You!

HEALTHY HABITS

WORD FOR THE DAY

SLEEP　　**MOVE**　　**RELAX**　　**CONNECT**

★

MY STRENGTHS

Situations cannot be changed,
but how you view them can.

DATE

TODAY I AM GRATEFUL FOR...

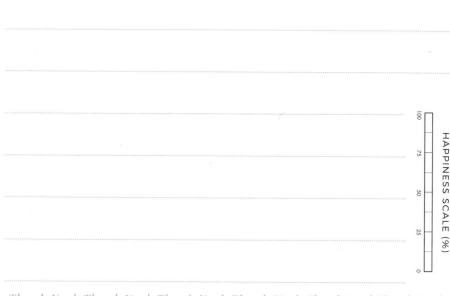

HAPPINESS SCALE (%)

100

75

50

25

0

Thank You! Thank You! Thank You! Thank You! Thank You! Thank You!

HEALTHY HABITS

SLEEP   **MOVE**   **RELAX**   **CONNECT**

WORD FOR THE DAY

POSITIVE AFFIRMATIONS

I AM

Write and mail a letter to a loved one.

TODAY I AM GRATEFUL FOR...

HAPPINESS SCALE (%)

100

75

50

25

0

Thank You! Thank You! Thank You! Thank You! Thank You! Thank You!

HEALTHY HABITS

SLEEP   **MOVE**   **RELAX**   **CONNECT**

WORD FOR THE DAY

I AM

POSITIVE AFFIRMATIONS

YOU ARE
A UNIQUE,
AMAZING BEING
THAT DESERVES
TO BE HAPPY.

inspiration

Deep belly, or diaphragmatic, breathing, is one of the easiest resilience building tools out there.

HOW TO BREATHE

We do it all day every day, so what is the value in breathing, other than the obvious?! Well that comes from its impact on your sympathetic nervous system, which is otherwise known as your fight or flight response. When you are stressed you experience it physically – your heart rate increases to get blood pumping to your muscles, you sweat to cool down, you release adrenaline to increase strength and speed, your breathing gets faster and shallower to get fresh oxygen in quickly and your immune and digestive functions decrease to conserve energy.

These are all great things if you are running away from a sabre-toothed tiger, but less helpful when you are just trying to get through the day and struggling to wind down or focus on a specific task. That's where diaphragmatic breathing comes in. Your breathing rate is the only part of your sympathetic nervous system response that you can actively control. And when you bring your breathing rate down, it, in turn, switches everything else off. By changing your breathing pattern you can calm and slow down your heart beat, helping you to shift out of a stressful, emotional state. How amazing is that?!!

SO, HOW DO YOU DO IT?

START BY BREATHING IN THROUGH YOUR NOSE FOR A COUNT OF 4 SECONDS. HOLD FOR 1 COUNT AND THEN BREATHE OUT FOR A COUNT OF 4 SECONDS, LONGER IF POSSIBLE. AND REPEAT.

Make sure your breath is filling your diaphragm first, rather than your chest. You can check this by placing a hand on your belly and a hand on your chest. You want your bottom hand to move first and further.

Start by doing this for short periods of time whenever you are feeling stressed and then build it into your everyday practice. Ideally, you're aiming for 4+ minutes a day and extending your breath to 7+ seconds.

GET FAMILIAR WITH THIS BREATHING TECHNIQUE AND START
BUILDING IT INTO YOUR DAILY PRACTICE. USE THE HEALTHY HABIT
TRACKER ON YOUR JOURNAL PAGES TO TRACK YOUR TIME FOR
RELAXING. WAS IT BAD, OK OR GOOD?

RELAX

USE DEEP BREATHING TO RELAX AND MANAGE EVERYDAY STRESS

Progressive muscle relaxation is a technique that builds on diaphragmatic breathing and aims to strengthen the connection between your mind and your body. By building this connection you can better understand and respond to stress in the body. Whether it's tight shoulders, restless legs, or a clenched jaw – we all hold tension in our bodies and by targeting these areas you can reduce the stress signals being sent back to your brain.

To do this on your own, take a few minutes to settle your breathing and then focus on a group of muscles or a part of your body and actively release any tension you find there. Some people like to start at the feet and move upwards. If you want someone else to do the talking for you there are lots of apps and audio files out there that can guide you through the process. Experiment, find the right voice, accent, style, flow for you otherwise you might just find yourself getting distracted! By noticing where you hold tension, you bring awareness to that area and may find you are more active in trying to release the tension.

** PERFECT FOR BEDTIME OR IF YOU WAKEUP AND ARE FINDING IT HARD TO GET BACK TO SLEEP **

USE GRATITUDE AS YOUR SECRET WEAPON

When you are using your deep breathing try focusing your attention in the area of your heart. Here are two simple steps to help with your heart focus using the Quick Coherence® Technique from the HeartMath® Institute.

STEP 1.

Focus your attention in the area of the heart. Imagine your breath is flowing in and out of your heart or chest area, breathing a little slower and deeper than usual.

STEP 2.

Make a sincere attempt to experience a regenerative feeling such as appreciation or care for someone or something in your life.

Think of a time you felt good inside, and mentally go back to that moment or place and try to re-experience the feeling. The key is to focus on something you truly appreciate – laughing with friends, a special moment with a loved one or seeing a beautiful sunset... recreate that feeling, that radiates from your heart when you are experiencing true love and appreciation. Some people call it a "Warm Fuzzy" feeling. This technique, based on research done at the HeartMath Institute, helps you neutralise the stress* and brings the head and heart into sync.

Quick Steps: Heart-Focused Breathing; Activate a positive or renewing feeling.

** PERFECT FOR WHENEVER YOU RECOGNISE YOUR ENERGY BEING DRAINED. TAKE TWO OR THREE BREAKS EACH DAY **

*Research from The Heartmath Institute www.heartmath.org/research/
HeartMath is a registered trademark of Quantum Intech, Inc. Go to www.heartmath.com/trademarks

Quiet your mind, engage your five senses and give your attention to the here and now.

PRACTISING MINDFULNESS

Stress and anxiety make you feel unhappy and make life less enjoyable, as well as having a huge impact on your physical health. Practising mindfulness mediatation helps with self-regulation, emotional regulation, memory, learning, empathy, pain tolerance, and complex thinking to name a (very cool) few.

MINDFULNESS HAS TWO PARTS...

Purposefully paying attention to the present moment AND accepting what you experience without judgement.

You can practice mindfulness by paying close attention to your breathing (diaphragmatic breathing of course! See previous page) especially in those moments when you realise you are stressed or angry. Noticing what you are seeing, hearing, smelling, feeling – internally and externally. These are things we don't usually pay conscious attention to. Understand and accept that what you think and feel at any given time is momentary and does not define you (see also Managing Emotions on page 34). This is an incredibly powerful idea.

** CHECK OUT THE APPS SMILING MIND AND HEADSPACE FOR MINDFULNESS MEDITATIONS **

TRY SOME COLOURING IN...

Settle into the rhythm of the activity and take time to appreciate how it makes you feel.

Colouring in is a form of mindfulness that calms your mind and occupies your hands. Experts* say focusing your attention on simple tasks that require repetitive motion can act as a type of meditation. Thus, concentrating on something like colouring in can help to replace negative thoughts and create a state of peace in your mind, as you are forced to focus on the present and hence block out negative or intrusive thoughts. It can also serves as a relief from the stress and anxiety of our rushing modern world.

So put away your phone, turn off the TV, grab some coloured pencils and take some time out to colour in the pages included in this journal. See how calm and mindful you become.

*Research from the University of British Columbia and the Chemnitz University of Technology (2014)

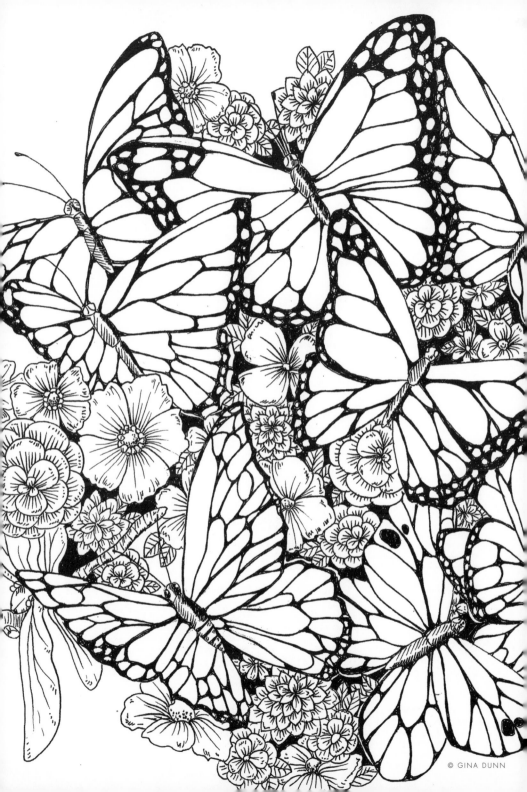

© GINA DUNN

Try mindful eating

We know that mindfulness is the process of giving our full attention to the present moment, but have you ever tried it while you are eating? Try giving your full attention to your food. Start with giving your full attention to your food choices and your appetite, it is easy to prepare our meals on autopilot! Make sure to sit down with out any distractions (easier said than done, right!), taste your food, really savour the flavour and texture. Be deliberate in what you choose to put into your mouth next, really notice your thoughts and physical experience with each mouthful. Try the chocolate meditation below.

CHOCOLATE MEDITATION

Sit comfortably, away from distractions.

Take a piece of your favourite chocolate (or treat) into your hand.

Now look at it.

Notice its weight and texture.

Look at its colour.

Notice how you really want to put it in your mouth.

Is your mouth watering?

Now smell it.

Have you noticed how it smelt before?

Now put it slowly into your mouth.

Let it sit on your tongue.

Notice the flavour.

Is it changing as it melts?

Is the flavour different to what you first thought?

Hold it on your tongue for as long as you can.

How does it feel?

NOW EAT IT!

** WHEN YOU OPEN THE FRIDGE OR PANTRY ASK YOURSELF IF YOU ARE REALLY HUNGRY. AUTOMATIC EATING BECAUSE YOU ARE BORED, OR CONDITIONED TO EAT AT A CERTAIN TIME, MEANS YOU MAY MAKE CHOICES THAT DON'T REALLY SATISFY OR NOURISH YOU. TRY EATING AT LEAST ONE MEAL MINDFULLY EACH WEEK **

PERSONAL CHALLENGE
Invite someone over for dinner.

TODAY I AM GRATEFUL FOR...

HAPPINESS SCALE (%)

100
75
50
25
0

Thank You! Thank You! Thank You! Thank You! Thank You! Thank You!

HEALTHY HABITS

SLEEP　　　**MOVE**　　　**RELAX**　　　**CONNECT**

WORD FOR THE DAY

POSITIVE AFFIRMATIONS

I
AM

Remember to always be kind.

DATE

TODODAY I AM GRATEFUL FOR...

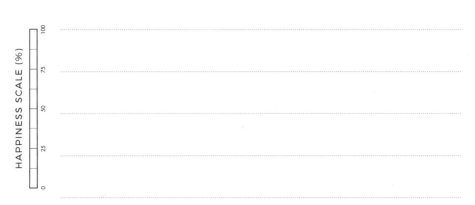

HAPPINESS SCALE (%)

100

75

50

25

0

Thank You! Thank You! Thank You! Thank You! Thank You! Thank You!

HEALTHY HABITS

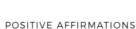

| SLEEP | MOVE | RELAX | CONNECT |

WORD FOR THE DAY

I AM

POSITIVE AFFIRMATIONS

I matter! I am worth it!

·············
DATE

WHAT WENT RIGHT THIS WEEK....

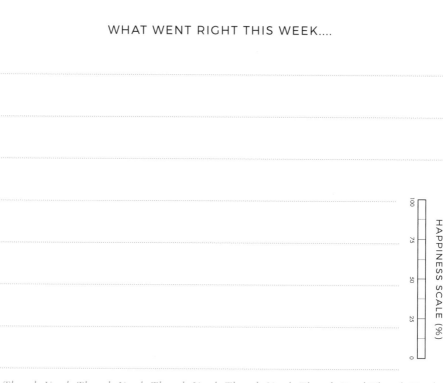

HAPPINESS SCALE (%)

100

75

50

25

0

Thank You! Thank You! Thank You! Thank You! Thank You! Thank You!

HEALTHY HABITS

SLEEP   **MOVE**   **RELAX**   **CONNECT**

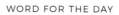
WORD FOR THE DAY

MY STRENGTHS

Let someone in front of you in line.

TODAY I AM GRATEFUL FOR...

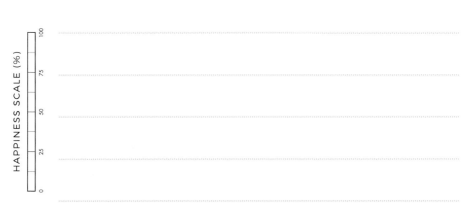

HAPPINESS SCALE (%)

100

75

50

25

0

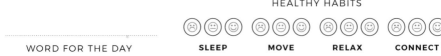

Thank You! Thank You! Thank You! Thank You! Thank You! Thank You!

HEALTHY HABITS

SLEEP MOVE RELAX CONNECT

WORD FOR THE DAY

I AM

POSITIVE AFFIRMATIONS

POSITIVE AFFIRMATION

What I want, wants me.

TODAY I AM GRATEFUL FOR...

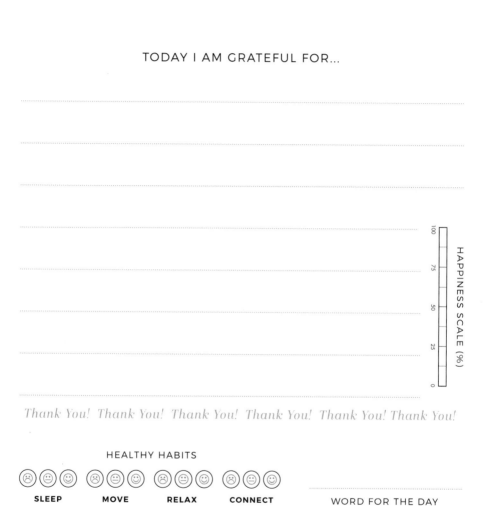

HAPPINESS SCALE (%)

100
75
50
25
0

Thank You! Thank You! Thank You! Thank You! Thank You! Thank You!

HEALTHY HABITS

☹ ☺ ☺   ☹ ☺ ☺   ☹ ☺ ☺   ☹ ☺ ☺

SLEEP   **MOVE**   **RELAX**   **CONNECT**

WORD FOR THE DAY

POSITIVE AFFIRMATIONS

I
AM

Mindfully breathe for five minutes.

DATE

TODAY I AM GRATEFUL FOR...

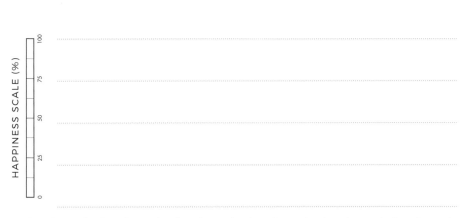

HAPPINESS SCALE (%)

100

75

50

25

0

Thank You! Thank You! Thank You! Thank You! Thank You! Thank You!

HEALTHY HABITS

WORD FOR THE DAY

SLEEP   **MOVE**   **RELAX**   **CONNECT**

I
AM

POSITIVE AFFIRMATIONS

DATE

POSITIVE AFFIRMATION

I am so grateful everything is working out perfectly.

TODAY I AM GRATEFUL FOR...

HAPPINESS SCALE (%)

100 75 50 25 0

Thank You! Thank You! Thank You! Thank You! Thank You! Thank You!

HEALTHY HABITS

SLEEP **MOVE** **RELAX** **CONNECT**

WORD FOR THE DAY

POSITIVE AFFIRMATIONS

I AM

*Thank someone who has
helped you at some point.*

DATE

WHAT WENT RIGHT THIS WEEK....

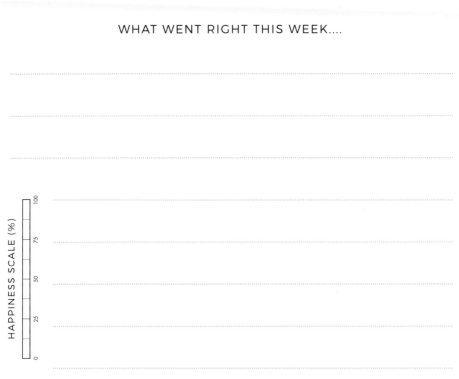

HAPPINESS SCALE (%)

100

75

50

25

0

Thank You! Thank You! Thank You! Thank You! Thank You! Thank You!

HEALTHY HABITS

WORD FOR THE DAY

SLEEP   **MOVE**   **RELAX**   **CONNECT**

MY STRENGTHS

Surround yourself with
people who lift you up.

DATE

TODAY I AM GRATEFUL FOR...

HAPPINESS SCALE (%)

100

75

50

25

0

Thank You! Thank You! Thank You! Thank You! Thank You! Thank You!

HEALTHY HABITS

SLEEP   **MOVE**   **RELAX**   **CONNECT**

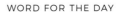

WORD FOR THE DAY

POSITIVE AFFIRMATIONS

I
AM

Hide a love note in
your partner's wallet.

....

DATE

TODAY I AM GRATEFUL FOR...

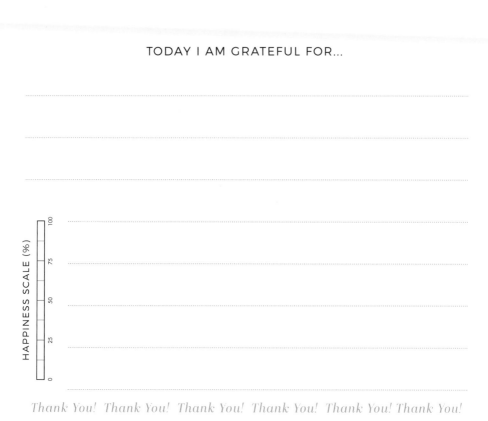

HAPPINESS SCALE (%)

100

75

50

25

0

Thank You! Thank You! Thank You! Thank You! Thank You! Thank You!

HEALTHY HABITS

WORD FOR THE DAY

SLEEP · MOVE · RELAX · CONNECT

I AM

POSITIVE AFFIRMATIONS

....

DATE

Make yourself a vision board
to manifest the life you want.

TODAY I AM GRATEFUL FOR...

HAPPINESS SCALE (%)

100

75

50

25

0

Thank You! Thank You! Thank You! Thank You! Thank You! Thank You!

HEALTHY HABITS

SLEEP   **MOVE**   **RELAX**   **CONNECT**

WORD FOR THE DAY

POSITIVE AFFIRMATIONS

I
AM

If it doesn't scare you, your
dream isn't big enough.

DATE

TODAY I AM GRATEFUL FOR...

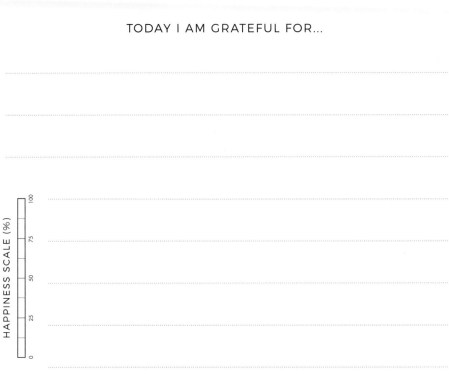

HAPPINESS SCALE (%)

Thank You! Thank You! Thank You! Thank You! Thank You! Thank You!

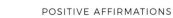

HEALTHY HABITS

| SLEEP | MOVE | RELAX | CONNECT |

WORD FOR THE DAY

I
AM

POSITIVE AFFIRMATIONS

Extraordinary things are coming my way.

....
DATE

WHAT WENT RIGHT THIS WEEK....

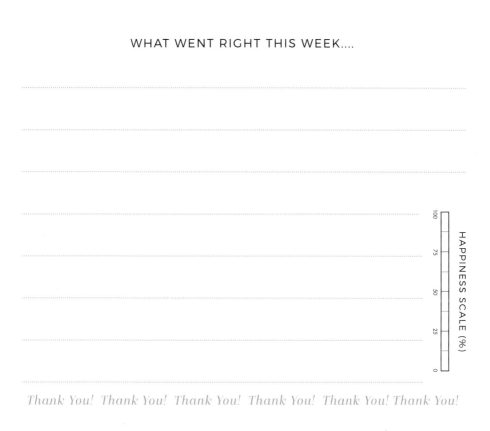

HAPPINESS SCALE (%)

100
75
50
25
0

Thank You! Thank You! Thank You! Thank You! Thank You! Thank You!

HEALTHY HABITS

SLEEP   **MOVE**   **RELAX**   **CONNECT**

WORD FOR THE DAY

MY STRENGTHS

Tell someone how grateful you are of them.

TODAY I AM GRATEFUL FOR...

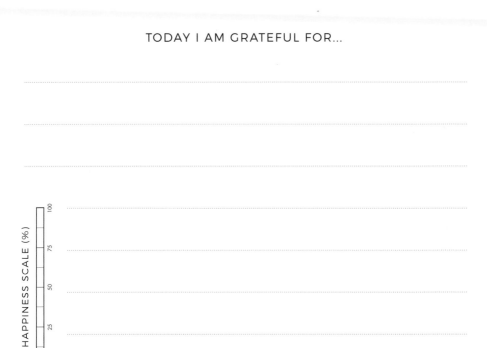

HAPPINESS SCALE (%)

100

75

50

25

0

Thank You! Thank You! Thank You! Thank You! Thank You! Thank You!

HEALTHY HABITS

SLEEP MOVE RELAX CONNECT

WORD FOR THE DAY

I AM

POSITIVE AFFIRMATIONS

*Flip those negative
thoughts into positive ones
and change your world.*

TODAY I AM GRATEFUL FOR...

HAPPINESS SCALE (%)

100

75

50

25

0

Thank You! Thank You! Thank You! Thank You! Thank You! Thank You!

HEALTHY HABITS

SLEEP　　**MOVE**　　**RELAX**　　**CONNECT**

WORD FOR THE DAY

POSITIVE AFFIRMATIONS

I
AM

Even bad days hold magical moments.

DATE

TODAY I AM GRATEFUL FOR...

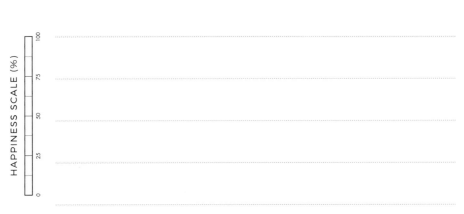

HAPPINESS SCALE (%)

100

75

50

25

0

Thank You! Thank You! Thank You! Thank You! Thank You! Thank You!

HEALTHY HABITS

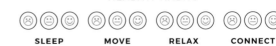

WORD FOR THE DAY

SLEEP **MOVE** **RELAX** **CONNECT**

I
AM

POSITIVE AFFIRMATIONS

TODAY I AM GRATEFUL FOR...

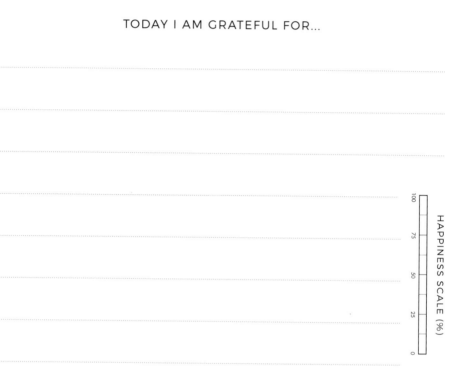

HAPPINESS SCALE (%)

100

75

50

25

0

Thank You! Thank You! Thank You! Thank You! Thank You! Thank You!

HEALTHY HABITS

SLEEP   **MOVE**   **RELAX**   **CONNECT**

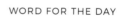

WORD FOR THE DAY

POSITIVE AFFIRMATIONS

I
AM

I am everything I ever wanted to be.

DATE

WHAT WENT RIGHT THIS WEEK....

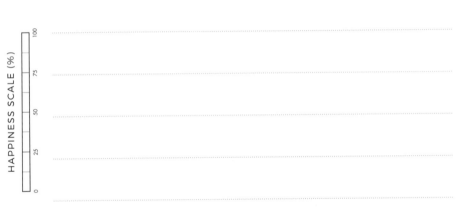

HAPPINESS SCALE (%)

100

75

50

25

0

Thank You! Thank You! Thank You! Thank You! Thank You! Thank You!

HEALTHY HABITS

SLEEP   **MOVE**   **RELAX**   **CONNECT**

WORD FOR THE DAY

MY STRENGTHS

TODAY I AM GRATEFUL FOR...

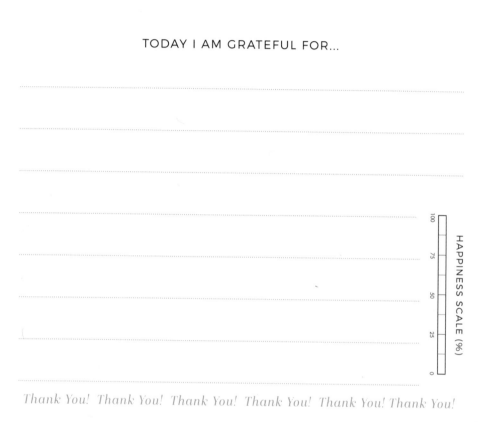

HAPPINESS SCALE (%)

100

75

50

25

0

Thank You! Thank You! Thank You! Thank You! Thank You! Thank You!

HEALTHY HABITS

SLEEP　　**MOVE**　　**RELAX**　　**CONNECT**

WORD FOR THE DAY

POSITIVE AFFIRMATIONS

I
AM

Pay for someone's parking.

TODAY I AM GRATEFUL FOR...

HAPPINESS SCALE (%)

100

75

50

25

0

Thank You! Thank You! Thank You! Thank You! Thank You! Thank You!

HEALTHY HABITS

 SLEEP   **MOVE**   **RELAX**   **CONNECT**

WORD FOR THE DAY

I AM

POSITIVE AFFIRMATIONS

TODAY I AM GRATEFUL FOR...

HAPPINESS SCALE (%)

100

75

50

25

0

Thank You! Thank You! Thank You! Thank You! Thank You! Thank You!

HEALTHY HABITS

SLEEP   **MOVE**   **RELAX**   **CONNECT**

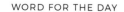

WORD FOR THE DAY

POSITIVE AFFIRMATIONS

I AM

PERSONAL CHALLENGE
Say "please" and "thank you"
and really mean it.

DATE

TODALY I AM GRATEFUL FOR...

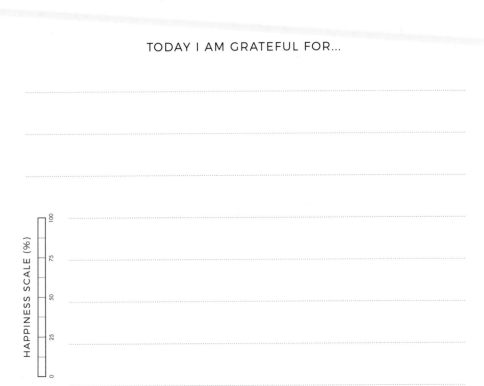

HAPPINESS SCALE (%)

100

75

50

25

0

Thank You! Thank You! Thank You! Thank You! Thank You! Thank You!

HEALTHY HABITS

WORD FOR THE DAY

SLEEP **MOVE** **RELAX** **CONNECT**

I
AM

POSITIVE AFFIRMATIONS

Find something to believe in.

DATE ....

WHAT WENT RIGHT THIS WEEK....

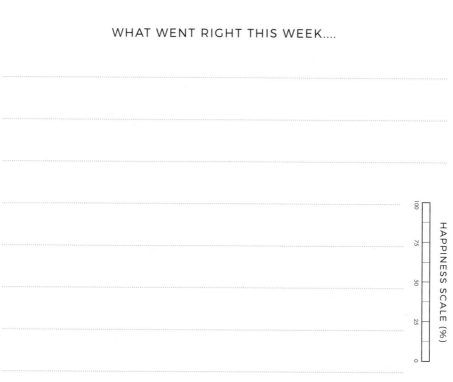

HAPPINESS SCALE (%)

100

75

50

25

0

Thank You! Thank You! Thank You! Thank You! Thank You! Thank You!

HEALTHY HABITS

SLEEP **MOVE** **RELAX** **CONNECT**

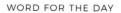

WORD FOR THE DAY

MY STRENGTHS

Hug a tree and give thanks for
the oxygen it provides you and
the beauty it shares.

DATE

TODAY I AM GRATEFUL FOR...

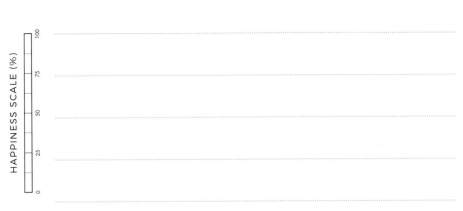

HAPPINESS SCALE (%)

100

75

50

25

0

Thank You! Thank You! Thank You! Thank You! Thank You! Thank You!

HEALTHY HABITS

SLEEP   MOVE   RELAX   CONNECT

WORD FOR THE DAY

I
AM

POSITIVE AFFIRMATIONS

LITTLE ACTS
OF KINDNESS
TOWARDS
OTHERS FEEDS
YOUR SOUL.

inspiration

Regardless of your age, or level of fitness, making time in your day for exercise can provide some serious benefits to your mental health.

FAST MOVEMENT

While pounding the pavement for hours might not be realistic or motivating for some, the physical and mental benefits of exercise that lifts your heart rate into what's known as the 'cardio zone' are well researched and hard to ignore. Many studies show that regular physical activity is correlated with improvement in clinical depression and anxiety, mild to moderate depressive symptoms, insomnia, and resilience under stress. People who become or remain physically fit or active are less likely to develop clinical depression.

WHY YOUR BRAIN LOVES EXERCISE

Moderate to high intensity exercise triggers a number of different chemical and hormonal changes in your brain, including: the release of endorphones that dull the sensations of pain; the release of serotonin that enhance your mood; increased blood flow that improves oxygen delivery and waste removal; the release of dopamine that improves motivation and learning; hormone release that protects the brain from degeneration; and the release of norepinephrine that improves attention and concentration.

This is why exercise has been shown to be effective as a treatment for depression (alongside therapy and medication). The end result of all these processes is a happier, healthier, more focused you.

CREATE AN ACTION PLAN

Making a commitment to exercise is sometimes easier said than done, so if you are struggling for motivation try creating an action plan. Your plan will include identifying what exercise you will do, when you will do it, where you will do it, how often you will do it and, most importantly, identifying the barriers, or excuses you put in place to not follow through and creating a contingency plan to manage those barriers or any other issues that may arise.

Make sure to pay particular attention to the reasons you give yourself for not doing it. By identifying our limiting or negative thoughts we are able to challenge them much more effectively.

** THE AIM IS TO GET YOUR HEART PUMPING SO TRY THESE IDEAS: CYCLING, BRISK WALKING, SWIMMING, CROSS-FIT, DANCING, SKIPPING, HIGH INTENSITY INTERVAL TRAINING, HULA-HOOPING, ROWING, USING AN ELLIPTICAL TRAINER, TRAMPOLINING **

EXERCISE ACTION PLAN

WHAT:

....

WHEN AND
HOW OFTEN:

....

WHERE:

....

WHAT ARE MY BARRIERS/EXCUSES?
e.g. I don't have time, the weather is bad.

....

....

....

....

WHAT IS MY CONTINGENCY PLAN?
e.g. get up earlier, keep spare running shoes at work, have a running buddy

....

....

....

....

The power of moving slow is the ability to combine many different tools that kick start our neurochemical and hormone processes.

SLOW MOVEMENT

For many of us, a yoga, tai chi or pilates class can be a much more appealing option than a crossfit one. Less sweat, less strain, and a little more relaxation? While the differences in exertion level are more obvious, the reason we find it so much more relaxing may be less so. The power of gentler types of exercise comes from their ability to combine many of the different tools we have talked about already.

BREATH

There is a focus on controlled, diaphragmatic breathing. We know that this is a key tool in reducing our body's stress response. See page 122.

MINDFULNESS MEDITATION

The soothing music, the soft lighting, the fixed gaze or closed eyes, the focus on where your body is in space. These are all designed to create focus points to draw your attention away from your internal thoughts and are key elements of mindfulness practice. See page 124.

MUSCLE RELAXATION

The process of gently moving and stretching muscles in a controlled way that aims to strengthen the mind-body connection. It releases tension and brings awareness to areas of our body that are carrying stress.

GET OUTSIDE AND MOVE

The benefits of slow movement include lower heart rate and blood pressure, increased muscle relaxation, and breathing capacity, as well as improvements in perceived stress, depression, anxiety, energy, fatigue, and well-being.

Try going for a walk outside, in the bush or at the beach, for 20-30 minutes a day. it will make you feel more revitalised and energetic, and less tense and angry. This is because of the reasons mentioned above, and also because exercise increases endorphines and reduces the level of stress hormones in your body. Walking in nature or urban green space, rather than the city, has even more benefits. It reduces your heart rate and increases heart-rate variability. Researchers believe the mood benefits of exercising in nature can last long after you finish.*

** YOGA, IN PARTICULAR, IS ONE TYPE OF SLOW MOVEMENT THAT IS SUPER EFFECTIVE IN REDUCING SYMPTOMS OF STRESS AND EMOTIONAL DISTRESS **

*Barton, J. and Pretty, J. (2010) What is the best dose of nature and green exercise for improving mental health? A multi-study analysis *Environmental Science & Technology*, 44(10) 3947-3955

Five amazing reasons you need to do sun salutations

1. It is easy to do! You don't have to be a yoga expert to learn this simple sequence of poses.

2. It increases your energy circulation– your lungs, digestive system, as well as muscles and joints will all benefit.

3. It lengthens and tones your muscles AND mind – continuous practice will bring more strength, flexibility, and tone to your muscles as well as relaxing your mind.

4. It allows you to experience moving meditation – concentrating on your breathing provides a bridge between the body and the mind, allowing you to be present, in turn reducing stress and anxiety.

5. The Sun Salutation is a gesture of respect and gratitude to the sun, use each round as a dedication to one thing you are grateful for, and soon you will feel the uplift in your mood and spirit!

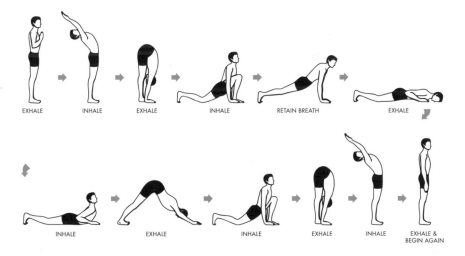

BUILD SLOW MOVEMENT INTO YOUR DAILY PRACTICE AND USE THE HEALTHY HABIT TRACKER ON YOUR JOURNAL PAGES TO TRACK HOW MUCH YOU MOVE EACH DAY.

MOVE

I am enough.

DATE

TODAY I AM GRATEFUL FOR...

HAPPINESS SCALE (%)

100

75

50

25

0

Thank You! Thank You! Thank You! Thank You! Thank You! Thank You!

HEALTHY HABITS

WORD FOR THE DAY

SLEEP   MOVE   RELAX   CONNECT

I AM

POSITIVE AFFIRMATIONS

DATE

Life is so precious but that gets lost in the mundane. Try to remember just how special life is.

TODAY I AM GRATEFUL FOR...

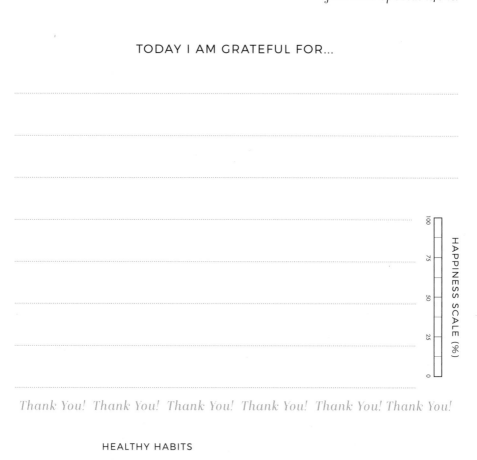

HAPPINESS SCALE (%)

100

75

50

25

0

Thank You! Thank You! Thank You! Thank You! Thank You! Thank You!

HEALTHY HABITS

SLEEP   MOVE   RELAX   CONNECT

WORD FOR THE DAY

POSITIVE AFFIRMATIONS

I AM

Say something kind to yourself.

TODAY I AM GRATEFUL FOR...

HAPPINESS SCALE (%)

100

75

50

25

0

Thank You! Thank You! Thank You! Thank You! Thank You! Thank You!

HEALTHY HABITS

WORD FOR THE DAY

SLEEP　　**MOVE**　　**RELAX**　　**CONNECT**

I
AM

POSITIVE AFFIRMATIONS

DATE

*Everything that we do, and
everyone that we meet, is put in
our path for a purpose.*

WHAT WENT RIGHT THIS WEEK....

HAPPINESS SCALE (%)

100
75
50
25
0

Thank You! Thank You! Thank You! Thank You! Thank You! Thank You!

HEALTHY HABITS

SLEEP   MOVE   RELAX   CONNECT

WORD FOR THE DAY

MY STRENGTHS

*There are so many reasons
to be happy today.*

SMILING IS CONTAGIOUS

We are all connected, so what we feel affects the people around us.

Smile at a stranger you pass on the street. If you make eye contact, they will likely smile back. This is called mirroring and is an unconscious, automatic response. It takes conscious effort to not smile back at someone smiling at you.[*]

Did you know that smiling makes you more attractive to others, as well as appear more trustworthy and generous?[**] Plus research shows smiling may increase lifespan, lower stress hormones and blood pressure.

Facial muscles send messages that modify the area of the brain that affect emotions and smiling stimulates those feel-good areas of the brain more than chocolate and money.[***]

[*]Sonnby-Borgström, M. (2002). Automatic mimicry reactions as related to differences in emotional empathy. *Scandinavian Journal of Psychology*, 43: 433-443.
[**]Golle, J., Mast, F. W., & Lobmaier, J. S. (2014). Something to smile about: The interrelationship between attractiveness and emotional expression. *Cognition & Emotion*, 28(2):298-310
[***]R. D. Lane & L. Nadel *Cognitive Neuroscience of Emotion*. Oxford University Press (2000).

DATE

Find time today for some slow movements like yoga.

TODAY I AM GRATEFUL FOR...

HAPPINESS SCALE (%)

100
75
50
25
0

Thank You! Thank You! Thank You! Thank You! Thank You! Thank You!

HEALTHY HABITS

😟 😐 🙂   😟 😐 🙂   😟 😐 🙂   😟 😐 🙂

SLEEP　　**MOVE**　　**RELAX**　　**CONNECT**

WORD FOR THE DAY

POSITIVE AFFIRMATIONS

I AM

I am beautiful, I am strong, I am happy.

DATE

TODAY I AM GRATEFUL FOR...

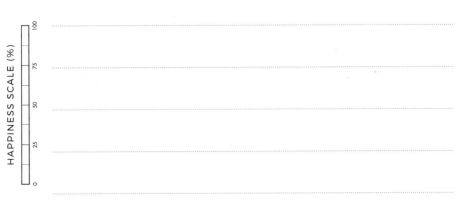

HAPPINESS SCALE (%)

100

75

50

25

0

Thank You! Thank You! Thank You! Thank You! Thank You! Thank You!

HEALTHY HABITS

| SLEEP | MOVE | RELAX | CONNECT |

WORD FOR THE DAY

I
AM

POSITIVE AFFIRMATIONS

....

DATE

TODAY I AM GRATEFUL FOR...

....

....

....

....

....

....

....

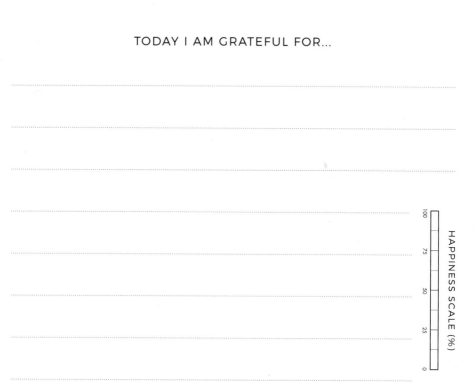

HAPPINESS SCALE (%)

100
75
50
25
0

Thank You! Thank You! Thank You! Thank You! Thank You! Thank You!

HEALTHY HABITS

SLEEP   **MOVE**   **RELAX**   **CONNECT**

....

WORD FOR THE DAY

POSITIVE AFFIRMATIONS

I
AM

....

....

Offer to carry someone's bags
or unload their groceries.

DATE

TODAY I AM GRATEFUL FOR...

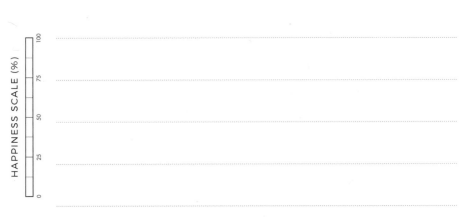

HAPPINESS SCALE (%)

Thank You! Thank You! Thank You! Thank You! Thank You! Thank You!

HEALTHY HABITS

SLEEP   MOVE   RELAX   CONNECT

WORD FOR THE DAY

I
AM

POSITIVE AFFIRMATIONS

Be grateful for everyday things.

DATE

WHAT WENT RIGHT THIS WEEK....

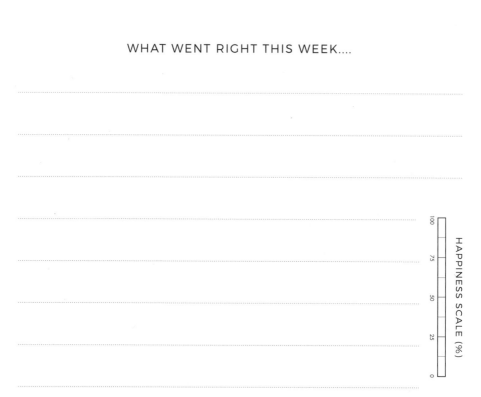

HAPPINESS SCALE (%)

100
75
50
25
0

Thank You! Thank You! Thank You! Thank You! Thank You! Thank You!

HEALTHY HABITS

SLEEP   **MOVE**   **RELAX**   **CONNECT**

WORD FOR THE DAY

MY STRENGTHS

I am a work in progress, always
evolving into a better version.

DATE

TODAY I AM GRATEFUL FOR...

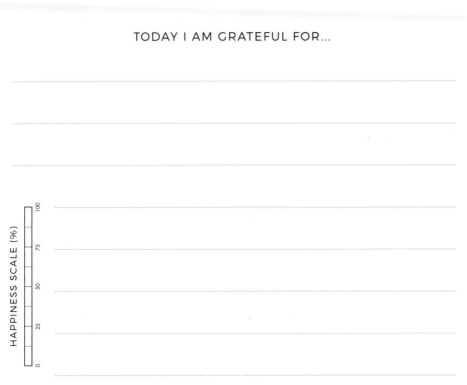

HAPPINESS SCALE (%)

100

75

50

25

0

Thank You! Thank You! Thank You! Thank You! Thank You! Thank You!

HEALTHY HABITS

WORD FOR THE DAY

SLEEP **MOVE** **RELAX** **CONNECT**

I AM

POSITIVE AFFIRMATIONS

*How can you understand
your soul, if you never spend
any time listening to it.*

DATE

TODAY I AM GRATEFUL FOR...

HAPPINESS SCALE (%)

100

75

50

25

0

Thank You! Thank You! Thank You! Thank You! Thank You! Thank You!

HEALTHY HABITS

SLEEP　　**MOVE**　　**RELAX**　　**CONNECT**

WORD FOR THE DAY

POSITIVE AFFIRMATIONS

I
AM

I can do this!

DATE

TODAY I AM GRATEFUL FOR...

HAPPINESS SCALE (%)

100

75

50

25

0

Thank You! Thank You! Thank You! Thank You! Thank You! Thank You!

HEALTHY HABITS

WORD FOR THE DAY

SLEEP **MOVE** **RELAX** **CONNECT**

I
AM

POSITIVE AFFIRMATIONS

DATE

*It is ok to have lazy days or time
to unwind and relax. Let the guilt go.*

TODAY I AM GRATEFUL FOR...

HAPPINESS SCALE (%)

100

75

50

25

0

Thank You! Thank You! Thank You! Thank You! Thank You! Thank You!

HEALTHY HABITS

SLEEP   MOVE   RELAX   CONNECT

WORD FOR THE DAY

POSITIVE AFFIRMATIONS

I
AM

You are in charge of how you feel, so choose what makes you happy.

DO SOMETHING NICE FOR SOMEONE ELSE

Giving to others releases endorphins that activate the parts of our brains associated with trust, pleasure and social connection.

Spending money or doing something for others leads to higher levels of happiness, and increases the chance that we'll be generous in the future. Plus when others see us being kind, they also get a hit of endorphins and are more likely to then go out and do something kind themselves.* This creates a positive feedback loop of generosity and happiness. The trick is to do something without being asked.

Kindness also contributes to good social relationships and therefore kind people experience more happiness and have happier memories. The experience of positive emotions and increased social interactions create an upward spiral of well-being.**

*Schnall, S., Roper, J. and Fessler, D.M.T. (2009) Elevation leads to altruistic behavior. *Psychological Science.* 21(3) 315–320
**Otake, K., Shimai, S., Tanaka-Matsumi, J., Otsui, K., & Fredrickson, B. L. (2006). Happy people beome happier through kindness: A counting kindnesses intervention. *Journal of Happiness Studies.* 7(3), 361–375.

WHAT WENT RIGHT THIS WEEK....

....

....

....

....

....

....

HAPPINESS SCALE (%)

100
75
50
25
0

Thank You! Thank You! Thank You! Thank You! Thank You! Thank You!

HEALTHY HABITS

SLEEP   **MOVE**   **RELAX**   **CONNECT**

....

WORD FOR THE DAY

MY STRENGTHS

....

....

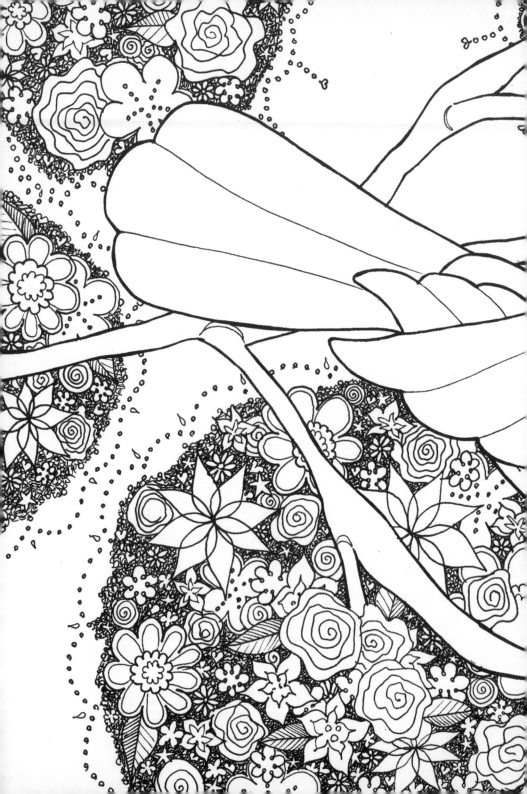

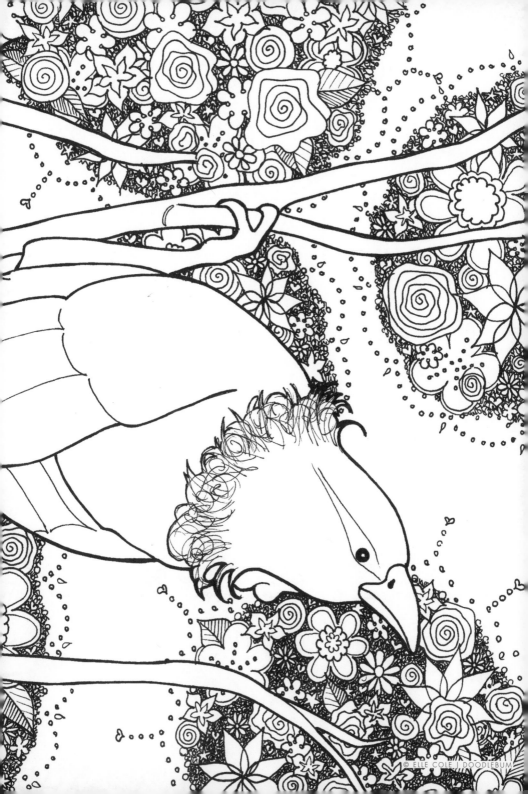

DATE

TODODAY I AM GRATEFUL FOR...

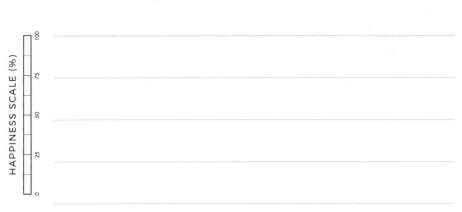

HAPPINESS SCALE (%)

100

75

50

25

0

Thank You! Thank You! Thank You! Thank You! Thank You! Thank You!

HEALTHY HABITS

WORD FOR THE DAY

| SLEEP | MOVE | RELAX | CONNECT |

I
AM

POSITIVE AFFIRMATIONS

······
DATE

TODAY I AM GRATEFUL FOR...

HAPPINESS SCALE (%)

100
75
50
25
0

Thank You! Thank You! Thank You! Thank You! Thank You! Thank You!

HEALTHY HABITS

SLEEP　　**MOVE**　　**RELAX**　　**CONNECT**

WORD FOR THE DAY

POSITIVE AFFIRMATIONS

I AM

175

Go for a swim today.

TODAY I AM GRATEFUL FOR...

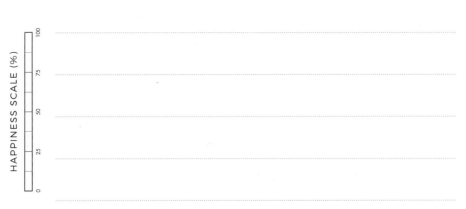

HAPPINESS SCALE (%)

100

75

50

25

0

Thank You! Thank You! Thank You! Thank You! Thank You! Thank You!

HEALTHY HABITS

WORD FOR THE DAY

SLEEP **MOVE** **RELAX** **CONNECT**

I AM

POSITIVE AFFIRMATIONS

We are all made of the stars,
so remember to shine.

DATE

TODODAY I AM GRATEFUL FOR...

HAPPINESS SCALE (%)

100

75

50

25

0

Thank You! Thank You! Thank You! Thank You! Thank You! Thank You!

HEALTHY HABITS

SLEEP   **MOVE**   **RELAX**   **CONNECT**

WORD FOR THE DAY

POSITIVE AFFIRMATIONS

I AM

*Find something to get
passionate about.*

WHAT WENT RIGHT THIS WEEK....

HAPPINESS SCALE (%)

100

75

50

25

0

Thank You! Thank You! Thank You! Thank You! Thank You! Thank You!

HEALTHY HABITS

SLEEP   MOVE   RELAX   CONNECT

WORD FOR THE DAY

MY STRENGTHS

PERSONAL CHALLENGE
*Go somewhere you have
never gone before.*

TODAY I AM GRATEFUL FOR...

HAPPINESS SCALE (%)

100

75

50

25

0

Thank You! Thank You! Thank You! Thank You! Thank You! Thank You!

HEALTHY HABITS

SLEEP   MOVE   RELAX   CONNECT

WORD FOR THE DAY

POSITIVE AFFIRMATIONS

I
AM

Go for a run or fast walk.

DATE

TODAY I AM GRATEFUL FOR...

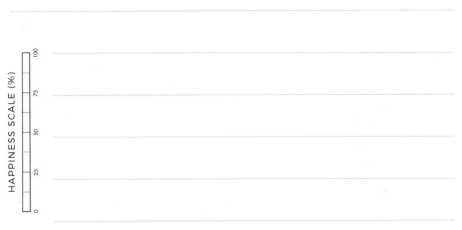

HAPPINESS SCALE (%)

100

75

50

25

0

Thank You! Thank You! Thank You! Thank You! Thank You! Thank You!

HEALTHY HABITS

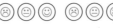

SLEEP   **MOVE**   **RELAX**   **CONNECT**

WORD FOR THE DAY

POSITIVE AFFIRMATIONS

I
AM

You can bear almost anything
if you have a reason to.

....

DATE

TODAY I AM GRATEFUL FOR...

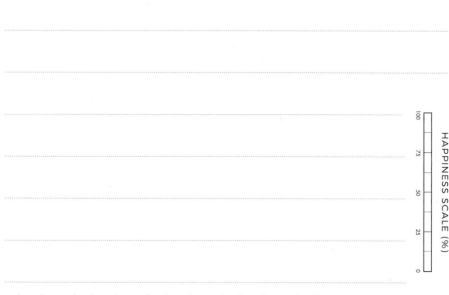

HAPPINESS SCALE (%)

100

75

50

25

0

Thank You! Thank You! Thank You! Thank You! Thank You! Thank You!

HEALTHY HABITS

SLEEP   **MOVE**   **RELAX**   **CONNECT**

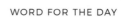

WORD FOR THE DAY

POSITIVE AFFIRMATIONS

I
AM

*Beauty is everywhere, open
your eyes and you will see it.*

DATE

TODAY I AM GRATEFUL FOR...

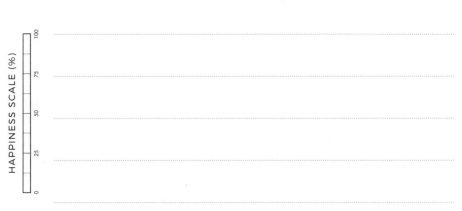

HAPPINESS SCALE (%)

100

75

50

25

0

Thank You! Thank You! Thank You! Thank You! Thank You! Thank You!

HEALTHY HABITS

SLEEP MOVE RELAX CONNECT

WORD FOR THE DAY

POSITIVE AFFIRMATIONS

I
AM

*Find an opportunity to give
someone a compliment.*

DATE

WHAT WENT RIGHT THIS WEEK....

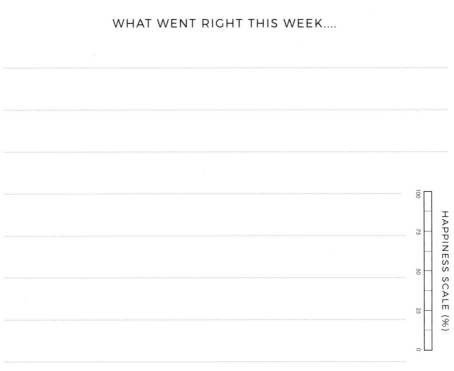

HAPPINESS SCALE (%)

100

75

50

25

0

Thank You! Thank You! Thank You! Thank You! Thank You! Thank You!

HEALTHY HABITS

SLEEP   **MOVE**   **RELAX**   **CONNECT**

WORD FOR THE DAY

MY STRENGTHS

Help others find the positive.

....

DATE

TODAY I AM GRATEFUL FOR...

....

....

....

HAPPINESS SCALE (%)

100

75

50

25

0

....

....

....

....

Thank You! Thank You! Thank You! Thank You! Thank You! Thank You!

HEALTHY HABITS

WORD FOR THE DAY

SLEEP   **MOVE**   **RELAX**   **CONNECT**

I AM

POSITIVE AFFIRMATIONS

....

....

*Retrain your mind to see
the good in everything.*

DATE

TODAY I AM GRATEFUL FOR...

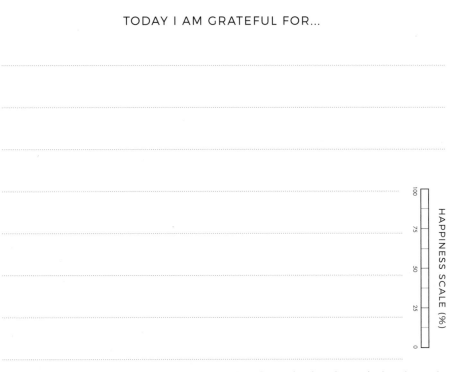

HAPPINESS SCALE (%)

100

75

50

25

0

Thank You! Thank You! Thank You! Thank You! Thank You! Thank You!

HEALTHY HABITS

SLEEP **MOVE** **RELAX** **CONNECT**

WORD FOR THE DAY

POSITIVE AFFIRMATIONS

I
AM

Get started today,
there is no better day.

DATE

TODAY I AM GRATEFUL FOR...

HAPPINESS SCALE (%)

100

75

50

25

0

Thank You! Thank You! Thank You! Thank You! Thank You! Thank You!

HEALTHY HABITS

WORD FOR THE DAY

SLEEP   MOVE   RELAX   CONNECT

I AM

POSITIVE AFFIRMATIONS

Walk barefoot on the grass.

DATE

TODAY I AM GRATEFUL FOR...

HAPPINESS SCALE (%)

100

75

50

25

0

Thank You! Thank You! Thank You! Thank You! Thank You! Thank You!

HEALTHY HABITS

SLEEP   **MOVE**   **RELAX**   **CONNECT**

WORD FOR THE DAY

POSITIVE AFFIRMATIONS

I AM

Five lessons learned...

Identify the top five challenges you faced over the last six months.
By identifying your challenges, how you handled them, and what
strengths you used, it will help you face challenges in the future.

INSPIRATION
Wake up, live your life,
be awesome.

INSPIRATION
*Follow the positive flow,
not the negative one.*

We believe everyone deserves to live a fulfilling, content and happy life.

This Resilient ME® journal will help you to build resilience and boost happiness so you can create a life worth living.

GRATITUDE (NOUN)
The quality of being thankful; readiness to show appreciation for and to return kindness.
OXFORD UNIVERSITY PRESS: THE OXFORD DICTIONARY

Many people find that making a choice to practice gratitude is one of the most useful things they can do to build resilience. It can help you bounce back from stressful events, and deal with adversity, by helping you to focus on the good things already in your life. It also helps to stop you keeping your emotions and thoughts on the inside.

The Resilient ME® journal by AwesoME Inc® not only teaches you how to get the most out of your gratitude practice, but also provides an insight into many tools and techniques, based on the best psychological research, to help you build resilience. By challenging negative thought patterns, creating a growth mindset, focusing on your strengths, setting goals, creating meaningful connections, and maintaining healthy habits you can live the most fulfilling life possible. The detailed eCourse, the resilience tools are based on, can be found at www.theResilienceToolkit.com

AWESOME inc.®

For more information about AwesoME Inc®, our awesome products for adults, teens and children, more research, amazing articles PLUS how to buy a new Resilient ME® journal go to:

WWW.THEAWESOMEINC.CO.NZ (NZ/AU)
WWW.THEAWESOMEINC.COM (USA)